Praise for *The Hunger Fix*

"In *The Hunger Fix*, Dr. Peeke tackles one of the greatest health problems of our day with startling new insights. She addresses food addiction at its root cause rather than simply providing a diet that leaves people hungry and dissatisfied. *The Hunger Fix* is a must-read for anyone who wants to end overeating and food obsessions once and for all."
—Norman E. Rosenthal, MD, clinical professor of psychiatry, Georgetown University Medical School, and author of the *New York Times* bestseller *Transcendence: Healing and Transformation Through Transcendental Meditation*

"In *The Hunger Fix*, Dr. Peeke shows how the foods we eat can directly alter brain chemical messengers and why some find it so challenging to just say 'no' to sugary, fatty foods. More important, she offers solutions and tools to counter the vicious cycle of food addiction."
—Michael W. Smith, MD, medical director, chief medical editor of WebMD.com

"*The Hunger Fix* presents research that is shockingly undeniable— food addiction is real! But there's hope for those struggling with hunger and overeating. Dr. Peeke's easy-to-follow plan will help readers rewire their brains and transform their bodies permanently. If you've tried everything and failed, this book is your savior."
—Chuck Runyon, founder and CEO of Anytime Fitness and author of *Working Out Sucks!*

"*The Hunger Fix* provides people of all sizes, shapes, and ages the opportunity to cast aside self-destructive behaviors and instead get high on Healthy Fixes. We couldn't agree more that injecting joy and fun into daily physical activity generates the real reward we're all hungering for as we seek long-term happiness and wellness!"
—Kathie and Peter Davis, cofounders of IDEA Health and Fitness Association

"In this groundbreaking book, Dr. Peeke successfully links the new science of addiction with the practical realities of our primal drives for hunger and appetite. Through this mind-body connection, *The Hunger Fix* offers a simple lifelong weight management and lifestyle solution that touches all aspects of how we think, eat, and play."
—Paul Terpeluk, MD, MPH, medical director, Employee Health, Cleveland Clinic

"Diets are based on denial and deprivation—they create a vicious cycle that leaves dieters feeling addicted to food. In *The Hunger Fix*, Dr. Peeke explains the science and biochemistry associated with addiction and food binges and offers simple eating steps for people who feel hopeless and out of control."
—Nancy Clark, MS, RD, CSSD, sports nutritionist and author of the bestselling *Nancy Clark's Sports Nutrition Guidebook*

"In *The Hunger Fix*, Dr. Peeke guides readers through the groundbreaking new science of food addiction, helping to explain how their reward systems can be altered by exposure to certain foods. After identifying the challenge, she provides an accessible, practical, science-based strategy to manage cravings and addictive habits for the long term."
—James O. Hill, PhD, cofounder, National Weight Control Registry, and executive director, Anschutz Health and Wellness Center, University of Colorado

The Three-Stage Detox and
Recovery Plan for Overeating
and Food Addiction

THE
Hunger
FiX

PAM PEEKE, MD, MPH, FACP

with Mariska van Aalst

RODALE.

Rodale books may be purchased for business or promotional use or for special sales. For information, please write to: Special Markets Department, Rodale Inc., 733 Third Avenue, New York, NY 10017.

Printed in the United States of America

Rodale Inc. makes every effort to use acid-free ⊗, recycled paper ♻.

Book design by Amy King

Library of Congress Cataloging-in-Publication Data is on file with the publisher.
ISBN-10: 1–60961–452–6 hardcover
ISBN-13: 978–1–60961–452–2 hardcover

Distributed to the trade by Macmillan

2 4 6 8 10 9 7 5 3 1 hardcover

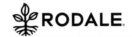

We inspire and enable people to improve their lives and the world around them.
rodalebooks.com

To anyone, of any age or size, who has ever felt helpless, hopeless, and defeated by their relationship with food. You *can* achieve the dream of lifelong control over your lifestyle choices. You *can* achieve optimal health.

Also to the extraordinary men and women who shared their stories throughout this book. Each of them has offered priceless words of wisdom as well as the hope that you, too, can discover their secret to success: *What you truly hunger for is not found in the fridge nor the pantry.* Instead, as one man said so eloquently, it's the peace that comes from learning to live your life to the fullest.

Find your true hunger and therein lies your real reward—control, peace, and joy. They did it. So will you.

Contents

Foreword by Tara Costa

MANY OF YOU MAY KNOW ME FROM THE HIT reality television show *The Biggest Loser*. I was on the show in Season 7, competing with my friend Laura. We were former models.

My brief time on the ranch at the *Biggest Loser* was just one stop on my weight-loss journey. You see, before applying to the *Biggest Loser,* I had what Dr. Peeke calls an "EpiphaME"—a moment that rang my bell and made me realize I needed to change my life.

It was May 24, 2008, my best friend's Lauren's birthday. That night, I stood in front of a nightclub with a bunch of my friends. By all accounts, it should have been a fun and carefree night. We had two cabs full of beautiful girls, and Lauren knew a promoter, so everything was taken care of—no waiting on line, no paying for drinks. I remember thinking, "Wow, we are set! This night is going to rock!"

As we walked straight up to the door, I had a moment of nostalgia— I used to do this kind of stuff all the time in my past modeling life. This was *fun*, getting dressed up and going dancing!

The bouncer unlocked the red velvet rope and the first group of girls walked right in the club. Now it was time for the second group of girls, including me, to go in. Suddenly I felt intimidated and shied away in the back. I hadn't been clubbing for so long (and I looked a lot bigger now).

As we walked up to the rope, my friends were let in one after the other—boom, boom, boom. Then my worst nightmare came true. The bouncer let in *all* of my friends, then stopped me and locked the velvet rope! I'll never forget his words, "We're at capacity!"

My first thought was "Bullshit—that's what they say when *they don't want to let you in*." My second thought was "Get me the hell out of here." I was mortified and ashamed.

I weighed 316 pounds.

I got into the first cab that I could find and told the driver to drop me off on the corner of my block, even though I lived halfway down the street. You see, my local bodega was on that corner, and it had all my little food friends that medicated me through life's hard times.

The second I walked into that bodega, a strange calm came over me. It was as if my problem was solved. Before I knew it, I stood in front of my two best friends—Ben & Jerry. Now the important questions raced through my mind: New York Super Fudge Chunk? Chunky Monkey? Or Karamel Sutra! I no longer cared about the humiliating rejection I just faced, because now I had what I thought was my reward—but what Dr. Peeke calls my "False Fix."

The truth is, I am a food addict.

I didn't become 316 pounds overnight. Packing on the pounds was a process, one that, at times, I don't want to remember. But finally facing what got me there is what has helped me realize that I never want to be like that again—lost, dissociated from myself, and hungering for the lies and the quick fix of my food addiction.

I'm an emotional eater. Whether I was sad or extremely happy, it didn't matter—every emotion was registered as "hunger" and filled with food. And the fact that most of my family has weight issues, and the majority of them are still obese, certainly didn't help. Sunday dinners at Grandma's house had four courses! There was no getting up in the morning to take a walk. We were clued out.

I had horrendous habits—I lived from one False Fix to the next. I would order breakfast from McDonald's every morning. In New York City they deliver! (Shocking, right?) I would order dinner in the car heading home from work and would eat in bed every night. I was out of control, living in a food trance. Like any food addict, I had my favorite False Fixes: chicken Parmesan, Ben & Jerry's, Entenmann's Pop'ems, fried chicken, waffle fries with cheese, Famous Amos cookies.

After 9 months of appearing on *The Biggest Loser*, and subsequently doing a tremendous amount of work on three important areas—what Dr. Peeke terms Mind, Mouth, and Muscle—I realized I needed different outlets to help me handle my emotions and stresses and express all the feelings I'd been numbing with my False Fixes. At times I still find myself looking at the dessert table, wishing I could have it all. I realize now that's my "inner addict" speaking. It'll always be with me, but I've learned how to turn what used to be a screaming command to stuff my face into a controlled, barely audible whisper.

My life today is no longer spent obsessing about how I am going to get my 3 o'clock latte and cookies. I am fully into what Dr. Peeke describes as a Stage 3 Master Recovery: I have maintained 80 percent of my numeric goal for over a year, and I am no longer hungry for the False Fixes. I reject that False Hunger. Instead, I have keyed into my *real* hunger, the thing that drives me: *How I can help others embrace a healthy lifestyle?* Now that I have discovered my real hunger for a better life, I'm following through and completing a master's in physical education, working as a body appreciation coach, and serving as the founder/president of my Inspire Change Foundation.

I look at the reminders that my current body and life is what I want forever—photos of me finishing the New York marathon, and flying through the finish line at the Kona Ironman triathlon. I humbly accept the fact that I will never be cured of my food addiction, but I do believe that I can lead a life of recovery. Every day I have the power to make the right choice, for my mind, body, and spirit. My own personal slogan reflects Dr. Peeke's 24-hour rule perfectly: "Just For Today—I can."

Most of us do not understand that once we identify our true hunger, we can set the scope of our dreams—that no matter how powerful the influences are, we do not have to be trapped by our environments. This is something Dr. Peeke has been preaching for years.

I will never forget the day that I met Dr. Peeke. I was running in the *More* Women's Half-Marathon in New York City. I saw Dr. Peeke from afar—she was surrounded by a huge group of women, all standing in a circle, just laughing out loud! From that moment, I knew I had to meet her—I love being around people who make others laugh.

When the festivities of the night began, Dr. Peeke got up on stage to deliver her trademark "Go get 'em" prerace dinner keynote. Instantly I could see she was a woman with a commanding presence, a truthful force who was also extremely compassionate. And she was leading her own team of Peeke Performers in the half-marathon the next day. She's the doc who truly walks her talk. She never hesitated in accepting the offer to be on my foundation board alongside Lance Armstrong's Livestrong team. I am privileged to have Dr. Peeke on my board and, more important, to have her as a friend and mentor.

Take it from me—a fellow food addict. This book will help you rid yourself of the shame and blame that you might feel because of your addiction. It helps you to understand how to win the day-to-day battles so you can end the lifelong war with yourself, once and for all. This book can change your life, if you allow it. You *can* get better. You *can* feed your true hunger. You *can* do this. Now is your time. Let's get started on your road to recovery.

Introduction

Hand Over the Chocolate and Nobody Gets Hurt!

WHEN LIFE GETS HARD, IS YOUR FIRST IMPULSE to eat?

Does the mere mention of a food, or seeing it in a picture or on TV, trigger you to obsess about and crave it?

Do you stockpile "emergency" snacks in your desk, closet, or nightstand?

Do you have to know where your next meal or food source is at all times—or you feel nervous, panicky, or "off"?

In times of high emotion, do you sometimes find yourself eating even when you feel no physical hunger at all?

Do you sometimes feel as though you're never quite satisfied or full enough after eating? Do you need more and more of the same foods to experience the same pleasure you once felt from that food?

Do you obsess about scoring your next meal, or counting calories, to the point of distraction or ignoring other obligations in your life, including your family and health?

Do you ever avoid social situations because you feel out of control in the presence of certain foods and will overeat?

Does your relationship with certain foods cause you to have feelings of shame, guilt, disgust, or self-loathing?

Do you sometimes feel like you could manage anything in your life—just as long as you didn't have to control your eating and you were "allowed" to eat and weigh whatever you want?

Is food your best friend and your worst enemy?

Is food your drug of choice?

If these questions sound familiar, you may be a food addict.

It's not just your imagination: *Food addiction is real.* You may be shocked or even relieved to read that sentence. But in your struggles with food, you may be tussling with an addiction that science has finally proved is every bit as powerful and painful as one to cocaine, heroin, alcohol, or nicotine. And every bit as hard to break as a serious gambling problem or a compulsive need for sex. (And, sadly, every bit as devastating to your relationships, pocketbook, self-esteem—even your life.)

All of these substances and experiences trigger a release of dopamine, a brain chemical that makes us feel a brief burst of pleasure and satisfaction. While you may have enjoyed these experiences guilt-free at one point, now your body and brain *hunger* for them to give you that numbing release in times of stress, to help you cope, to allow yourself to escape, to try to "fix" your unpleasant feelings. Yes, you know consciously that this fleeting "high" of pleasure and satisfaction can't fix the root of the problem—yet you can't resist the temptation of scoring just one more "hit" before you resolve to buckle down. Repeat this pattern enough times, and any of these "False Fixes" become the problem in itself.

So you keep desperately searching for your next hit. You're not really hungry. Yet you feel a draw, a gnawing hunger for these False Fixes, and there never seems to be enough to satisfy you, to put a period at the end of your pleasure-seeking sentence. Repeated exposure to all of these substances and experiences has the power to physically alter the neural structure and chemistry of our brains. Depending on your genetic history and how you manage your living circumstances and stress levels, these neurologically toxic False Fixes can quickly exhaust and wipe out half the population of your brain's dopamine receptors, which in turn only increases your appetite for more and more of your favorite False Fix. A scoop of ice cream was once enough. Then the large bowl morphs into the pint, then the half gallon. Respond with a greater "dose," and more receptors dwindle away. Before you know it—even in as short a time as a couple of months— your brain's reward system can turn against you, making it a closed loop that demands more pleasure, feels less, and cares only about scoring more—the endless hunger for a higher high. Your health, career, relationships, happiness be damned—you must have your False Fix.

Really? Can an innocent little cookie or piece of cake or bag of chips be that toxic and destructive? Come on, we're not talking about heroin, for crying out loud. We've seen what so-called real addictions can do. They can lure talented artists like Amy Winehouse and Heath Ledger to early graves. They can send Lindsay Lohan to a jail cell or Charlie Sheen to the unemployment line. In comparison, food addiction triggers can *seem* completely innocent.

A candy dish on your co-worker's desk.

A cookie tray coming out of the oven.

A smell of popcorn at the movies.

A quick fast-food lunch on a busy day.

A plate of steaming pasta.

While these tempting foods may seem like simple treats to many, when you're struggling with food addiction, they can be as alluring and irresistible to you as a glass of wine is to an alcoholic or a crack pipe or a line of coke is to a drug addict. When you're struggling with False Fixes, you may go through your entire day strategizing about your next fix. You may be finishing one meal as you plan the next, or find your fingers hitting the bottom of the chip or pretzel bag without even realizing you've been mindlessly auto-eating. You may find it uncomfortable to drive down the street without pulling into the drive-thru, or to go through the checkout line without buying the Snickers, "just in case" you can't get food later, when you'll "need" it.

To make matters worse, you may feel ashamed of these thoughts and feelings. But though it may feel like it, you are far from alone—we are a nation at war with food addiction. Some food addicts are skinny, but quietly obsessed, trying desperately to keep themselves in line. Others are overweight or obese. The diabetes rate is skyrocketing. Kids in their early teens are developing high cholesterol and insulin resistance. Metabolic syndrome is now the norm, not the exception. While not everyone who is overweight or obese is a food addict, I'll wager that the majority are.

We've been fighting the battle of the bulge—and losing—for a long time now. And we can shout about "personal responsibility" until the cows come home. Yes, of course, everyone needs to take care of his or her health and well-being. But in the past several decades, the brain chemistry of children, men, and women has been going through drastic, self-destructive changes. And these food-addiction-driven alterations in gene expression are being passed from one generation to the next.

You can no sooner tell a food addict to just "eat less and move more" to solve his or her problem than you can tell a drug addict to just suck it up and quit. Nobody is ever going to convince me that the two-thirds of the people in this country who are overweight simply got that way due to laziness and lack of discipline. No one *chooses* to be fat—at least not consciously. Who in God's name would willingly choose to become society's biggest pariah?

Studies have revealed that, as a group, overweight people get fewer promotions, have less-satisfying relationships, and endure crushing depression and loneliness. And make way less money: One study found that obese women make about $16,000 less a year than thin women.[1, 2]

In a world that's becoming more sensitive to racial, gender, religious, and sexual differences every day, overweight people have become the last "safe" butt of cruel jokes, the whipping boys and girls for everything from high health care costs to plane crashes to global warming. So who in their right mind would *choose* to subject themselves to that?

No one would. But while we were all getting on with our lives, earning a paycheck, and just trying to get through the day, the modern convenience food supply has hijacked our reward system. Chronic exposure to processed foods—science-fair projects packed with sky-high salt, unhealthy fat, and refined sugars—have tapped into our most basic instincts, turning our neurochemistry, our brain tissue, even our very gene expression against us.

We are at a crossroads. The typical eat less, move more (ELMM) strategy doesn't address the unique mental, physical, spiritual, and biological hunger of food addiction. The days of throwing every overweight person on a 1,200-calorie diet are over.

We have to treat food addiction as we would any other life-threatening addiction—we have to resist addictive foods with every fiber of our being and recommit to that fight on a daily, hourly, minute-to-minute basis. Vigilance is imperative to the recovery process.

Alcoholics do it. Former smokers do it. Even heroin addicts do it. We applaud their efforts because we know how hard it is, once those addictions have taken control of their bodies, to have the strength to say no to that False Hunger for the fix every single day.

We have to look at losing excess body weight—and keeping it off—as a lifelong process of recovery that doesn't end but can get easier and easier—and more and more rewarding—the more we practice.

I'm not going to lie. Recovery from food addiction can be compli-cated. Hard-core drug addicts actually have it *easier* than people who struggle on their own with food addiction.

Why? Because drugs, cigarettes, and alcohol are not needed for survival. Once you get clean, *you never touch the substance again.* You are abstinent for the rest of your life. Your life then revolves around avoiding the persons, places, and things that will place you at high risk for relapse. You stick to safe environments and support sys-tems where it's unlikely you'll be exposed—what a relief! You don't ever have to nibble a little rock of crack at a Super Bowl party.

You don't pass by a vodka dispenser at every gas station and 7-Eleven.

You never walk down a grocery store aisle packed with loaded syringes of heroin.

You get off the stuff, tell yourself you'll never touch it again, and there's no gray area. Recovering drug addicts and alcoholics know what they have to do: Just say no. Steer clear. *Forever.*

The harsh reality with food addiction is that abstinence from all food is *not* an option. You must walk among your "drugs" every day of your life. You cannot escape them, no matter where you go. But I'm here to tell you, with my plan's simple tools and techniques, you can learn how to calmly and confidently enter any "dangerous" food situation and know that you'll walk out feeling proud and empow-ered instead of helpless, hopeless, and defeated.

And best of all—you'll enjoy the sensuous experience of eating delicious food *even more* than you do now. You'll appreciate flavors you never knew existed. You'll discover feelings in your body you didn't even know you could feel. You will not feel deprived at all—because you'll learn that deprivation is not the solution, it is the enemy. In fact, you know the secret to your success is to feel *extra* satisfied, in every way.

How will you do this? It's very simple.

How the Hunger Fix Works

You hunger for a better life, the freedom to do what you love and to enjoy and embrace every single moment. But you're stuck with a different hunger. A gnawing, craving, tearing-your-insides-out, desperate, and frantic search for just one more food fix. Just one. But the hunger is insatiable. It never ends. And it's standing in the way of your ability to live your life to the fullest.

There *is* a way to fix this addictive hunger. In *The Hunger Fix*, I'm going to show you how chronic exposure to your False Fixes has led to False Hunger. Your brain's reward center has been hijacked, leaving you with an itch you just can't scratch. Then I'll show you how to manage your own biology—reclaim your reward center, quell the cravings, free yourself from the viselike grip of your food addiction.

With *The Hunger Fix*, you'll learn to tap into your innate reward neurochemistry to work the way nature intended. Using the latest neuroscience research, I have developed a program that systematically addresses each facet of the powerful reward system, capitalizing on a specific sequence of natural triggers, to make the entire cascade of neurochemicals work *for* you instead of against you. The Hunger Fix plan puts the science on your side and teaches your brain to derive as much pleasure—and eventually more—from positive, life-affirming Healthy Fixes as it does from the negative, health-destroying False Fixes. The more you master the ability to swap good fixes for bad, the faster you reclaim total control of your brain and your body.

Believe it or not, eventually even the process of kicking a False Fix will become a reward in itself. Trust me—that deep feeling of satisfaction and mastery is more addictive than any plate of nachos or chocolate cake will ever be.

Let me be clear: The dopamine-driven neurochemical cascade of reward is a masterpiece of human survival machinery. In fact, the instincts behind the brain's reward system are likely the driver behind all of human evolution. The reward-driven brain propels us to love and reproduce, to feel curiosity and be motivated, to be creative, to innovate, to dream BIG. And while certain facets of modern living have hijacked this system to get us to consume more and more, we can at any moment revert to our body's natural state of being and use our God-given dopamine bliss for good instead of evil. We just need to know how.

The Hunger Fix is a three-stage lifestyle-makeover/weight-management plan that progressively alters the chemical balance, neuropathways, and genetic expression in your brain, so your body relearns how to get the dopamine rush you crave—without self-defeating patterns that keep you fat, broke, bored, and unhappy.

You will move through the three stages at your own pace. You may hit milestones at different times than other folks might, but you'll see (and definitely feel) results almost instantly. Addictions vary as much as people—some people can rein in their impulses and addiction with much greater ease than others. Cross-addictions (where people have more than one addiction) will intensify the food addiction. But whether you are skinny, slender, overweight, or obese, this plan honors everyone.

I'll give you as much structure or as much flexibility as you'd like: You can follow the eating plan to the letter, down to every bite for breakfast, lunch, dinner, and snacks—or you can mix and match your meals and your strategies to fit your own life. You can follow every tip and use every technique, or you can pick and choose the ones that speak directly to your core concerns. This plan must work for *you*—your life, your preferences, your needs, your hunger—because learning to adapt and adjust to whatever life throws at you without self-destruction is a core skill for all recovering food addicts.

The Hunger Fix plan teaches you:

- How to scientifically determine, once and for all, if you are a hard-core food addict
- How to identify and then abstain from your "bingeable" or False Fix foods

- How certain food nutrients and ingredients keep your dopamine levels elevated—such as the amino acids tyrosine and phenylalanine, catalyzed by vitamins and minerals like B_6 and zinc—and how to stock your kitchen with every possible source of these "safe high" micronutrients

- How meditation significantly helps to support food addiction recovery by healing the addiction-ravaged brain, growing brain cells to replace those lost to False Fixes, supporting recovery, and preventing relapse

- How every mental, nutritional, and physical activity choice you make is reflected in changes in how your very genes—the epigenome—communicate with the rest of your body to either help or hinder your detox and recovery

- How you can use specific low-sweat exercises to increase the body's production of brain-derived neurotrophic factor, or BDNF, a protein that stimulates new growth in several areas of the brain—including the areas best known for helping people stick to long-term goals

- How moderate exercise guards against dips in acetylcholine, a neurotransmitter essential to preventing relapse and "supersensitivity" to rebound cravings—so you'll start out slow and easy, building your physical endurance and strength

- Which rhythmic cardio activities warm up the hypothalamus and increase the brain's release of soothing, calming serotonin, nature's antidepressant

- Why "diets" that deprive the brain of natural reward and pleasure fail because they cause chronic elevations of cortisol (stress hormone), *creating* stress, the main driver of addiction—and how the Hunger Fix program completely sidesteps this extremely common pitfall with a primary focus on *satisfaction*

- How taking the *right* kinds of creative personal or professional risks can be the biggest dopamine high of all—and, when done correctly, a guaranteed way to keep weight off for life

- How to find your authentic, Healthy Hunger for a better life

Whether you're overweight or not, this plan will help you shed the mental weight and burden of food addiction. But if you *are* overweight, you'll also shed pounds and inches—an achievement that in the past might have prompted you to reward yourself with a manicure or a movie night for "a job well done." (Or even a food treat that would restart the cycle of addiction and self-destruction!) With *The Hunger Fix*, all food addicts will learn how to indulge themselves right away in an unlimited amount of dopamine boosters—*massage, dancing, sex, intellectual challenges, video games, public speaking, meditation, playing cards, arranging flowers, strolling in the woods, sleeping, drinking cold water, driving fast cars, even goal setting itself.* You'll learn how these immediate rewards guard against the hormonal supersensitivity that can lead to relapse. Plus, they simultaneously generate new dopamine receptors that increase the amount of delight you're able to wring out of every moment. You'll be having a blast!

Every step you take in the Hunger Fix program will yield new neural circuits in your ever-growing-and-changing brain. Every stage of your plan will make it progressively easier, more automatic, and immeasurably more pleasurable to have the body you want and the life that you've always dreamt of.

Are You with Me?

I've spent my entire career helping people navigate the health challenges of modern life. From my fellowship at the National Institutes of Health (NIH) to the publication of my *New York Times* best-selling books and through my academic writing and keynote, television and radio appearances, and magazine articles, I have brought cutting-edge science to bear on the immense challenges of weight management. I've always been about optimizing the quality, not just the quantity, of your body.

Yet, as you'll hear in Chapter 1, even I'm not immune to False Fixes. And neither is my family or most of my friends and colleagues—even world-renowned addiction and weight researchers. We all struggle with this issue to one degree or another. We've all tasted the waters of the sugary, fatty, salty foods foisted on us since childhood. It's a permanent memory in our bodies. There's no going back—only forward. Together, we are going to reclaim our reward systems and manage our weight and health without self-destruction.

I've taught thousands of people how to outrun the grasp of food addiction and open up their lives to a whole new chapter of empowerment, joy, mastery, and freedom from the grip of their False Fixes—and now I want to help you.

Let's do this.

CHAPTER 1

The Dopamine Made Me Do It!

THERE IS NOTHING BETTER THAN A FRIEND,
UNLESS IT IS A FRIEND WITH CHOCOLATE.
—ANONYMOUS

WE ALL HAVE ONE.

At least one.

A little darling. A best friend. A helper, a life raft.

An entrenched habit that's so comfortable, it feels like a hug or an island of calm.

A fix.

A fix starts simply enough. You think about doing something that you like to do—drink a mojito, or check your iPhone, or get it on with your boyfriend or girlfriend—and that thought lights up an entire dopamine-driven reward pathway in your brain.

You feel a rush of pleasure. You start thinking about when and how you are going to do that thing:

Is it happy hour yet?

Can I sneak a peek at my e-mail during this meeting?

Will he or she be around tonight? When are we going to connect?

Your brain becomes consumed by the drive to satisfy that urge. You try, but you just can't get it out of your head. You give in.

And then, as soon as you satisfy the raging hunger, bingo: You feel another rush. Your brain says, "Yeah! This is amazing. Bring it on. I want more."

You need your fix.

Most of the time, this neurological process is a good thing. Nature wants humans to stick around, so she uses this system to reward us for doing things that will ensure our survival—eating food, bonding with loved ones, having sex, making babies. Preferably as often as possible.

As a result, everything we do—from the time we wake up until we collapse into bed—is driven by reward. We're either getting reward in the short term (enjoying an hourlong massage) or in the long term (earning a college degree after studying for 4 years).

The reward can also be to avoid pain. I learned that as a little girl who didn't like to brush her teeth. After suffering through a cavity, I soon learned that my real reward was never seeing that dentist again.

This same reward system drives us to learn, to create, to innovate, to pursue our goals. But as a medical doctor specializing in metabolism and weight management, logging thousands of hours a year to educate the public about behavioral change, I've seen firsthand how the dopamine rush cuts both ways. The tremendous high you get from a run in the park or a hike to the top of a mountain can be powerful enough to change your life. But that healthy high occupies the same pathways, and can easily become confused with, the dopamine hit from a snort of cocaine or a puff of a cigarette. Clearly, not all rewards are created equal—and some can kill you.

In the past few years, I've started to see a growing manifestation of this double-edged sword in my own medical practice. More and more men and women are coming into my office desperate to find an answer to the same questions: Why can't I stop thinking about food? How can a cookie or plate of pasta or bag of chocolates have this kind of hold on me? I feel like a junkie!

As I listen to people's tortured stories of unbearable cravings, yo-yo dieting, weight obsession, and emotion-driven stress eating, I've seen a pattern emerge. Their pleas for help are no longer your standard "Gosh, I'd love to drop 10 pounds before the reunion" fare. Instead, these entreaties have become eerily similar to the cries for help from my patients with hard-core drug or alcohol addictions:

"I just need that sugar fix every afternoon. If I don't get it, I'll go crazy with withdrawal."

"I need a dose of pizza."

"Those Tostitos and dip are like crack to me—once I start, I just can't stop."

I started to realize that in more and more of my patients, these cravings are the result of a reward system gone awry. I had also reviewed the new science that shows the mere anticipation of that food-related dopamine high will cause the reward centers of the brain to light up like Times Square on New Year's Eve—the same as brain scans of cocaine addicts eager for their next fix. It doesn't take much to trigger this cascade of brain chemicals: A casually mentioned word, a picture in a magazine or on TV, or a smell from a bakery is all it takes to awaken the desperate cravings. That same insatiable drive for reward keeps all addicts pressing the dopamine accelerator, overriding their brain's normal "satisfaction" signals.

These dopamine-driven moments of pleasure start to accumulate. With constant practice, they progress to habits, carving deep neural pathways in the brain. With every repetition of the cycle, those pathways get stronger and healthier alternatives get pruned out to make way for these new, ultra-rewarding but unhealthy habits. A walk in the neighborhood with your best friend begins to pale in comparison with sitting in front of the TV and bingeing on bags of your favorite

I Need a Fix

Voices of Addiction[1]

On my blog on WebMD, I asked people to share their thoughts on food addiction—*is it real?* The answers were very telling. See if you can recognize yourself in any of these comments.

My addiction to ice cream and other sweets began in childhood. Celebrations were made with half pints of the hand-packed ice cream of our choice, which became an addiction to relieve grief, stress, and other emotions. Because after all—life is good with ice cream.

While I have been eating mostly healthy for 9 years, I still cannot have ice-cream-type things in my home—still a binge-type food. Why having it available sets me off, I have no idea.**—Jis4Judy**

For those whose recommendations include, "Well, just don't eat that," I wish it were that simple. It's like a smoker's need for cigs and an alcoholic's need for alcohol. If I have a lot of sweets available, I have a hard time not eating all of them. I keep it out of the house, except on special occasions.**—nursingbug**

I still struggle with the bread issue but am constantly re-focusing to look at what I really want: consistency, a comfortable weight, and peace of mind. When I eat binge foods, I switch into an addict, focused on the next fix. I hate that cycle, but not always enough to avoid it.**—init4life**

Of all the stresses I have subjected myself to in my life, I thought smoking was the worst. I never even thought I had an addiction to food!

When it was clear to me that I was as dependent on food as I was on smoking to get me through events, that's when I realized I was fighting one of the toughest enemies of all . . . me.**—mawsings**

My mother was an alcoholic. She did not eat much; she always felt she was competing for my father's attention, that she had to be thin. So she smoked and drank vodka. She hid the smoking from my father, and she would sneak her vodka on some occasions.

I was hiding foods because I was embarrassed by the size that I had become. Someone asked me why I just didn't stop eating the foods that I was gorging on. I could not do it at that time. I was not ready to change, and I had not hit my rock bottom.**—GoingForGoal** chips. This False Fix becomes the default, setting up a domino effect, constantly reinforcing itself.

See if this sounds familiar: Eat in bed, stay up too late, get rotten sleep. Feel like hell in the morning, reach for sugary, caffeinated foods to stay awake. Mindlessly seek the numbing of *"just one more* [candy/chip/cookie]." A glass of wine at dinner becomes three, and maybe even take a sleeping pill before bed to get "a good night's rest."

Without fully realizing it, many people have created a life of continuous, comfortable opportunities to "dope up" in front of the computer, in the doorway of the fridge, and on the couch. They are driven to repeatedly score hits of what I call "False Fixes"—anything (like food) that leads to short-term reward in association with self-destructive behavior, followed by feelings of guilt, shame, and defeat. In contrast, Healthy Fixes are productive, positive habits associated with feelings of pride, happiness, and achievement: the enjoyment of tasty, delicious whole foods, gardening on a sunny day, or taking a long walk with your best friend. When False Fixes prevail, Healthy Fixes are tossed aside. The seductive lies of the False Fixes now occupy center stage. In pursuit of each False Fix, you create self-defeating habits to support your habit. You start to set up rituals surrounding your bingeing. And voilà, you're ensnared in your own endless vicious False Fix–seeking cycle.

This phenomenon clearly isn't just in my practice. We can see ample evidence of what many False Fixes have created in society:

Right this second, 800,000 people are texting or chatting on cell phones while driving.

The average child spends 53 hours *a week* in front of some kind of screen.

The average American family carries almost $15,000 in credit card debt.

And now we see the emergence of food addiction, which is striking us at all ages: Toddlers' obesity rates have doubled in the past 30 years, and older kids' rates have tripled. Teens' rates almost *quadrupled.*

Half the population of the United States will be prediabetic or diabetic by 2020—an estimate that, as a devoted public health advocate and policy advisor, frightens me to the core. We've even made up new words—such as *diabesity*—to describe what we're becoming. Even men and women of average size who've never been seriously overweight can struggle with food obsessions and addictive behavior. Folks who have dropped weight and kept it off still continue to grapple with how to avoid their "crack." Food addiction does not discriminate—it can afflict people anywhere along their weight-management journey.

The Most Devious Fix of All

You can get high on dopamine in many different ways. Some fixes are productive, like going to the gym or reading the Sunday *New York Times*. These highs build you up—you come away from them feeling proud, fulfilled, and eager for more. These are Healthy Fixes.

A False Fix, by contrast, is destructive. You feel guilty, ashamed, and disappointed.

This is the last time. Never again. And I mean it.

But once the False Fix cycle is triggered, you feel like you don't have a choice.

Some False Fixes, like drugs, nicotine, and alcohol, are clearly addictive substances. And let's not forget sex and gambling. But food? Is it a federal offense to rip through an entire cheesecake? Will you be hauled off and convicted of a felony fat count?

For years, many of my colleagues refuted the fact that food can be "addictive." Yes, the research said that foods can be habit forming—but just on a behavioral level. There was no proven biological basis to believe otherwise. What people need is willpower! Hey, it's just a cookie, for crying out loud. Control yourself! Discipline!

Addiction researchers have long documented the danger of "real" drugs of abuse. Not only can you die from your meth addiction, this addictive substance directly changes the physical structure of your brain. As drugs hijack the pleasure system and wipe out dopamine receptors, the brain adapts and adjusts, creating a tolerance that demands ever more of its drug to get the same False Fix high. Eventually the addict has to have the substance to simply feel normal. He doesn't just want it; he needs it. He hungers for it.

At that point, all other healthy survival motivations—self-care, family, friends, career, sex, love—are cast aside in favor of scoring the drug. Researchers call this deadly change "motivational toxicity," which, in the case of hard drugs, can run its course pretty quickly: Basically, unless you get clean, you're looking at jail or even death.

Well, some experts would say, unlike heroin, meth, or crack, at least you can't die from OD'ing on Jamocha Almond Fudge—at least not immediately. So food wasn't considered a "real" addiction. It's never been taken seriously. Until now.

In the past couple of years, the entire medical field has started to shift. Researchers have uncovered irrefutable proof that food itself can, even under the strictest definitions, be considered a substance of abuse. Nora Volkow, MD, director of the National Institute of Drug Abuse (NIDA), has committed millions of dollars to studying the relationship between food and addiction.

Dr. Volkow is my hero. She has made it her professional mission to study how certain foods can hijack the brain's reward system. Beginning her odyssey in 2001, Dr. Volkow and her team used PET scans and radioactive chemicals that bind to dopamine receptors.[2] Their research revealed that obese people had far fewer dopamine receptors in the brain's striatum, the reward center, and therefore had to eat more to experience the same reward or high as average-weighted individuals.

In 2002, Dr. Volkow delved into the craving or "wanting" question. When people were exposed to their favorite treat foods but were not allowed to eat them, a tidal wave of dopamine surged through the striatum.[3] They said they "hungered" for their fixes. Yet they weren't hungry at all. This is exactly what happens in the brain of drug abusers after just watching a video of people using cocaine.

Since these landmark findings, numerous NIDA-funded studies published in gold-standard peer-reviewed journals such as *Nature Neuroscience* have proved that the brain is forever changed by this food addiction cycle of anticipation and reward. When rats are given free access to the kinds of "highly palatable foods" that we humans are surrounded with all the time—such as chocolate, cheesecake, bacon, sausage, and other fat and processed food treats—these foods change the structure of the brain the same way that cocaine does. Researchers from Yale University have used functional MRI (fMRI) studies to prove that both lean and obese women who test positive for addictive behavior around food show the exact same pattern of neural activity as a chronic drug abuser: very high levels of anticipation of their drug of choice—in this case, a chocolate milk shake—but very low levels of satisfaction after consuming them.[4]

The addiction develops like this: Think of a river during a flood. The water charges over the banks, taking down trees and houses along the way. Continued dopamine flooding in the brain works the same way. The pathway between the ventral tegmental and the nucleus accumbens areas of the brain floods with dopamine again and again. The brain think it has "too much" dopamine—so the brain attempts to compensate for this overabundance by battening down the hatches, decreasing the total number of dopamine receptors to lessen the amount of dopamine your brain absorbs. This "down regulation" decimates receptors in a variety of brain regions, particularly your limbic system, the site of motivation and emotions.

After this down regulation, your brain demands you eat greater and greater amounts of the same foods to elicit the same dopamine "rush." You have an insatiable hunger for more and more. But the sad irony is, the more you feed the craving with False Fixes, the less satisfaction you feel—because each time you flood the brain, additional receptors get wiped out. And the relentless hunger persists.

As these receptors disappear, the abilities of other parts of your brain to communicate with each other also take a hit. In 2008, Dr. Volkow published a study in which her team found that obese people who have fewer dopamine receptors also have less activity in their prefrontal cortex.[5] The prefrontal cortex, aka the PFC—the grown-up, responsible part of your brain that gets you to work on time and brushes your teeth and pulls your hand back from the dessert tray—gets cut off from all the action in the mesolimbic pathway. This is a double whammy: Not only do you have to eat more food to experience normal pleasure, but you also have a tougher time stopping once you do eat. The PFC might be shouting, "No! Don't eat it! You don't want to get diabetes!" but it's too late. Your brain has a permanent memory of your False Fix. All your limbic system can hear is "Carpe diem, baby! Screw everybody. Come on, it's just a cookie. Dig in!"

That's your "inner addict" speaking with that familiar "it's just a _____" seduction. Your command central, the PFC, is getting out-shouted and smacked down. This "delay discounting" tendency—ignoring the long-term ramifications of short-term pleasure—gets stronger and stronger as the limbic system's receptors dwindle and the communication channel with the PFC gets weaker and weaker. Instead of hearing the strong, stern voice of the PFC reminding you to stop, think, and be mindful, your reward system is deafened by the roar of immediate gratification.

Bang! The False Fix has won.

This is why stressing "moderation" to addicts is a moot point. While in full addiction mode, their PFC function is impaired. When the protective reasoning of the PFC is no longer part of the equation, the results can get ugly fast. Food addicts desperately hunger for their False Fix and will go to extraordinary lengths to make sure they can get their hands on it. They may spend much of their time thinking about food and withdrawing from other people in embarrassment to "do" their food in privacy.

Lab rats with unlimited access to a high-fat/high-carb diet almost eat themselves to death. They'll voluntarily opt to walk across an electrified plate and endure painful shocks in order to get their hit of junk foods. In one study, when rats had access to high-fat/high-carb food for only 1 hour of the day, they would consume 65 percent of their daily calories in one sitting, just continuously gorging until the food was removed from their grasp. But once the food was removed, they didn't simply shrug their rodent shoulders and turn back to regular chow. No, they withdrew and curled up into the fetal position, soothing themselves with nervous hand-wringing, becoming excessively twitchy and easily startled. They were hungry for their fix, and without it, they ended up with what's known in the addiction world as "the shakes."[6] They were mini-junkies coming off of the stuff, their drug, their crack.

When we've lost touch with our PFC and we are guided solely by ever-louder dysfunctional dopamine cravings for False Fixes, we are no different than those rats. I've seen it happen, again and again. My patients say things like, "Fresh-baked bread with big lumps of butter— it's like a drug to me. I can't stop eating it. Oh my God, my mouth is watering just talking about it. . . ."

Yep. That False Fix indeed won.

How Food Became a False Fix

We know the statistics: Worldwide, obesity has doubled in the past 30 years.[7] In 1980, one in six Americans was obese; today that number is one in three.

What the hell happened in those 30 years?

When researchers from the University School of Medicine in St. Louis first did a study of almost 40,000 people in the early 1990s, addictive genes appeared to have no impact on body weight. People were just as likely to be obese if they came from a family with addiction as if they didn't.

But when scientists did a follow-up study of 40,000 other people in 2001 and 2002, the picture was very different. Now people were 30 to 40 percent more likely to be obese if they had addiction in the family. For women, the chance was 50 percent greater.[8]

The huge upsurge in obesity in the last 30 years was not caused by evolutionary changes to the genome. The basic genetic makeup of humanity could not change that quickly. No, this explosive weight gain was caused by changes to the environment that *switch on* our individual genes.

The new science of epigenetics (*epi* meaning "around" and *genetics* referring to the study of genes) helps us understand how *any* environmental cue—any person, place, or thing—can influence how our genes are expressed. If you live and participate in an active social community, with plenty of fresh food and opportunities for fun exercise, the genes that control your weight can operate as nature intended, and you can more easily enjoy a fit and healthy body.

But if you skip your breakfast and drive your 30-mile commute and have a psycho boss waiting for you at the office, and you're not equipped with the right stress management strategies, your fight-and-flight genes will go into overdrive and hit total burnout. Your levels of acetylcholine and cortisol, stress hormones that trigger fat storage and cravings, go through the roof. To anesthetize the pain of your daily existence, you may dope up with continual False Fixes—often those conveniently available at the office vending machine or drive-thrus on your way home. This constant dependence on False Fixes not only thickens your waistline and changes your brain structure but also takes its toll on your genes, changing their expression to one supporting addiction—further reinforcing the cycle.

Here's another shocker. Think you're in the clear because your parents and grandparents lived long lives? Wrong. When you have continuously fallen prey to your False Fixes and the behavioral changes that support them, this changes your gene expression. And this altered gene expression is passed on to your children. Your food addiction becomes theirs.

Of course, this is not just happening to you. Just like in drug abuse epidemics, the combination of adverse living conditions plus increases in the *availability* and *concentration* of substances of addiction makes it easier for the environment to switch on those addictive genes.

Yale researcher Ashley Gearhardt likens this evolution in food availability and calorie concentration to the history of cocaine.[9] Once, the innocent coca plant leaves were merely chewed as part of South American religious rituals. Then, in the 19th century, coca started being processed into cocaine. A source of addiction for some, yes—but still restricted to a small part of the population.

Then, in the early 1980s, came an "innovation" in cocaine production: Low-quality cocaine was processed into a cheaper, more highly concentrated, more easily transported drug. Crack cocaine was born—as was, amid rising poverty and homelessness, the devastating crack cocaine epidemic of the mid- to late 1980s.

Now, says Gearhardt, take corn. Corn on the cob has always been a beloved seasonal staple of the American diet, at home on any picnic table. Then, in the late 1970s, due to the development of new fructose enrichment technology, corn started being processed into high fructose corn syrup, a cheap, highly concentrated, more easily transported source of sweetness than cane sugar. In the "fat-free" diet-obsessed years that followed, HFCS was added to hundreds and then thousands of inexpensive, heavily processed, widely available foods.

The result? From 1980 to 2009, our consumption of added sweeteners rose 40 percent.[10] Our intake of HFCS had risen from almost zero to 13.2 teaspoons *a day*.[11]

Gearhardt is not exaggerating when she says we are now experiencing something akin to that crack crisis. Surrounded on all sides by these concentrated sources of sugary, fatty, salty False Fix food rewards[12]—and aided and abetted by environmental toxins; car-bound, sedentary living and work spaces; disconnected communities; canceled recess; and the thousands of other 21st-century stresses to the genome—we now have an epidemic of food addiction, with the 24/7 False Fix lifestyle to support it. That is precisely why *The Hunger Fix* is not just about food addiction but instead about every element of your living that supports your food addiction habit.

Who's Your Sugar Daddy?

Some people are more vulnerable to all of life's False Fixes than others. Those who've endured a major trauma or abuse, have a family or personal history of addiction (often referred to as cross-addictions), or have suffered from depression, anxiety, or ADHD may have a higher predisposition—they may even start using their False Fixes simply to self-medicate. Some folks try to get clean, but their roommates, friends, or spouses remain blindly hooked, pushing False Fixes that trigger addictive cues, making a tough battle even tougher. Simply being female is a risk factor: A study in the journal *Biology of Sex Differences* found that female rats are more susceptible to addiction at smaller doses of drugs than male rats—which may help explain why women are more susceptible to emotional eating and binge eating.[13]

Fast-food restaurants don't hesitate to make hay with these weaknesses, in a big way. You've heard about those meat-bacon-meat-cheese-meat sandwiches, or stuffed-crust, deep-dish, sausage/ham/beef pizza. How many different ways can you infuse this one meal, one bite, with more fat, salt, and carbs? The sheer caloric density in one of these dishes causes a rush that normal foods cannot hope to equal. And all at a low, low price. It's a cheap "fix."

Take Blair River, the 575-pound spokesperson for the Heart Attack Grill, a restaurant in Chandler, Arizona, that prides itself on its meals of over 8,000 calories of "Double Bypass Burgers" and "Flat-Liner Fries."[14] A sign on the building reads, "Caution: This establishment is bad for your health." Their ads boast the tagline "Taste . . . Worth Dying For."

River recently died—at age 29.

The whole marketing hype behind the restaurant was poking fun at the so-called nanny state that doesn't believe in "personal responsibility" and just wants to legislate taste.

But given what we now know about the addictive nature of these types of foods, to food addicts, restaurants like the Heart Attack Grill have become something more like socially sanctioned, fully legal, heavily advertised crack houses.

Severely food-addicted people don't just think, "Oh, that looks tasty—I think I might have a nibble." Their addicted brains tell them, "You can't live without this food."[15] Sadly, like most intractable addicts—of nicotine, heroin, or cheese fries—the thing they couldn't live without is exactly what can kill them.

You don't have to be 575 pounds to be living the False Fix lifestyle. Whether it's 10 or 100 extra pounds, excess unhealthy body fat is the price people pay for their False Fix–driven lifestyles.

Easy for you to say, you might be thinking. *You're a doctor. And look at you—you've never had a weight problem.*

Oh, but I have. False Fixes emerged early in my own life. They packed an extra 50 pounds on me. And make no mistake—I know they're still right outside my door. But I was lucky enough, at a critical moment in my life, to realize the secret of staying one step ahead. Had I not learned these lessons early on, I shudder to think how my life could have taken a much different turn.

As you read my story, you'll see how I've benefited greatly from positive epigenetics. You'll see how life circumstances can profoundly change gene expression—and weight. You'll also learn that no matter how you got to where you are now, there is hope for a much better future.

My First Tangle with False Fixes

From the beginning, I was lucky. I was shielded from False Fixes as a kid. I was a tomboy growing up. Long and lean like my mom, muscular like my dad. Nobody in my family is obese. Genetically, I scored.

Living in San Francisco offered beautiful landscapes and countless hills. I was immersed in a healthy lifestyle. I went everywhere with my two older brothers—played basketball, swam laps. I also loved ballet: I dedicated myself to mastering pointe and could whip out some decent pirouettes. With five kids and thriving commercial real estate holdings, my mom and dad didn't have time to linger over preparing massive meals—we ate simply to give our bodies energy. Our attitude was: Food is fuel. We ate and moved on.

Then, when I was in my mid-teens, my younger sister contracted an autoimmune disease and became ill, and it seriously affected my entire family. As the older sister, it fell to me to take care of her and my kid brother while my mom and dad juggled their parenting and professional roles. Before my sister got sick, I would do my homework and play sports with my friends—that was about the extent of my responsibilities. But once the illness hit, my extracurricular activities fell by the wayside. I did paperwork after school so my mom could be with my sister. Or if Mom was needed at the office, I would go home, sit inside, and keep tabs on my sister as I stared forlornly out the window. I could hear my brothers yell around the neighborhood with their friends or run through the house on their way to a baseball game while I prepared dinner or washed the dishes.

I got mad. I felt frustrated, sad, and disconnected. But I kept it to myself. I knew my job. This was family.

A total bookworm, I started to retreat into books. If my body had to be at home, so be it—but my mind could wander the galaxy. On my way home from school, I would stop in a favorite bookstore on Market Street and pick up some science fiction or fantasy—*Dune, Lord of the Rings*. Then I'd hit the Woolworth's next door.

It started out with small bags of bridge mix. "Ten cents worth, please?" I'd ask, then tuck my treat into my bag and not take it out until I was home, under my covers, slipping into other worlds, making it all go away, if only for a short time. My athletic romps had transformed into rituals of withdrawal and chocolate-induced food comas.

Slowly, as the months went by, my candy bag got heavier. Ten cents became 20. A quarter pound, half a pound. Soon I became very comfortable saying, quite matter-of-factly, "A pound of bridge mix, please."

That candy had become my best friend. My False Fix. I didn't realize it at the time, of course, but I was medicating my feelings with food. The fat and sugar and salt of the chocolate, nuts, and caramel all swirled together in my brain, soothing my sadness, reinforcing the neural landmine I was planting each day that told me I "deserved" this treat—and rewarding me with a big rush of dopamine when I complied. I was gradually becoming addicted to the contents of those white Woolworth bags.

No one really noticed as the pounds came on. Kids at my nerdy-smart high school were wearing big, sloppy clothes around that time—stretched-out sweaters, cords, Empire-waist dresses worn over jeans. You could be 50 pounds overweight and no one would know. You could hide, and I did. Even from myself. I had completely disassociated my mind from my body. My mind cranked out the A's, but my body was a wasteland of food addiction.

When I got to college at Berkeley, it was worse. The coolest kids looked like Einstein on a bad day, with their hair flying all over the place, dressed in baggy jeans and sandals and burning the midnight oil at the library. No one looked good and no one cared. That was the stereotype, and I lived it. When I wasn't working, I was studying—overstudying.

Finally, right about the time my sister's situation calmed down, I began to come out of this fog. And as I did so, I noticed something interesting: My appetite began to decrease. I still felt the draw of the False Fix foods, but now that the severe stress was abating, I was finally awakening and becoming more aware of other forms of reward—namely, male attention.

One beautiful spring day in Berkeley, I went out with a really cool guy I met in physics class. (Okay, he was a bit of a nerd—surprise, surprise! I was, too!)

He was a sweetie. I desperately wanted to wear something that looked awesome. It was warm out, and for the first time, I realized I was uncomfortable wearing shorts in front of a guy. *What's that about?* I thought. I had no clue what size or shape I had become.

I put on a pair of brown corduroys that had worn thin. I thought I looked pretty good. We took a glorious walk through campus to the rose garden and back. We were just about to say good-bye—him to study, me to the lab, and then we were going to meet later that afternoon. He ran over to his car to get a book for me. I took one long stride toward his car and heard a rip: *My pants had split.*

Now the good news is, he never saw a thing because I had a sweater tied around my waist. But the pants split from the crotch, right down the middle section of my left thigh, and all the way to my knee. They were thin, overly washed pants—but that's not why they split. They split because they were way too tight on me.

I can, to this day, still hear the *rrrrip* of those pants splitting.

The good news is that we kept dating. But that experience was like someone took what I now call a "velvet sledge hammer" and whapped me across the head. Just rang my bell.

I went home, stood in front of the mirror, and said out loud, "My God, what happened to me? Where have I been? Where did I go?"

That was it. That was my moment, what I now call my "EpiphaME." I took the pants off and hung them in my closet, front and center. I saw them every time I opened that door—they were my humbler, a constant reminder to change my behavior and keep on track until I got where I wanted to be.

The very next thing I did was enroll in a ballet class. I still had my old ballet leotard and shoes. I had loved dance so much; it was painful to think about all the years I had missed. At my first class, I stared at myself in the mirror. *Who the hell is that?* I'd been wearing "hide it" clothes for so long, I was startled to see my body stripped down to a leotard and tights. Lumps and bumps abounded! I was awash in emotions—embarrassed, guilty, anxious, and angry. Determined, I pushed ahead and plunged into my first plié.

I was nervous. But my ballet skills started coming back.

And my appetite changed quickly. I became laser focused. *I am going to live now*, I thought. *I hunger for a better life. I am done with numb.*

It took me a number of months to regain my mental and physical strength, but I did that ballet class all the way up to pointe. I began to hike. Next thing you know, I was hiking at Lake Tahoe. I went Nordic skiing. I went surfing! I'd replaced my addiction hunger with a hunger to live my life to the fullest.

How long did all this take me? The morphing was extraordinary. I would say over the course of a year all of the extra 50 pounds dropped off. I had many things on my side. Genes. Early exercise that had built strong muscles waiting to be reawakened. A defiant determination and a passionate drive—a hunger—to succeed. And perhaps most important of all, I lived in Berkeley, California.

A co-op very close to where I lived had all kinds of nutrition education classes and fresh produce. Vegetarianism was taking off then, and the *Moosewood Cookbook* was all the rage. I taught myself to cook. I made big, delicious soups and invited tons of friends over to share.

I developed other new rituals. I would strap my bike on the back of my little Fiat convertible and drive up to Tilden Park behind the Lawrence Radiation Lab. I'd bike for miles and miles until I could see the Golden Gate Bridge and Sausalito and Mount Tamalpais. I would sit there and, for the first time, learned to meditate.

Right down my street, a brand-new restaurant showed up: Chez Panisse. Several times a week, I would eat an inexpensive, blindingly gorgeous lunch prepared by the renowned chef and my friend Alice Waters, in the very birthplace of the locavore, farm-to-table concept. I learned as a young woman just how good organic whole food tastes. My body started craving fruits and vegetables and whole grains and lean proteins.

Why am I telling you all this? Because now, as I look back, I can see now how incredibly *lucky* I was. What would've happened if I were living somewhere else, where junk food and smoking cigarettes were the norm? Consider what most college kids and graduate students do: Binge drink at frat parties. Smoke pot and get the munchies. Put on the "freshman 15"—or 40. Stress-eat their way through their dissertations.

Think back to your own late teens and early twenties, the time when we're starting to develop our own ways of interacting with the world. What did your life look like? If your habits were less than healthy, as they are for most of America, those neural patterns got set, hormone levels shifted, fat cells added—and those False Fixes got their claws into you that much further. Indeed, research has shown that children's tolerance for sugar can take a quantum leap forward within their first few years. You might not even get to middle school before your reward center has already set you up to become enslaved to False Fixes. Let alone all the lifestyle habits and epigenetic changes you'd already inherited from your parents. If your parents ate well and stayed active, they gifted you with a great start on life. On the other hand, if they were out of control, that got passed on as well.

I come to you "successfully fixed"—that is, addicted to a whole host of Healthy Fixes. I am a person who has kept a chunk of weight off for over 30 years. I've defied the odds. How? I altered my living environment to support my new healthy habits. I also realized that for the rest of my life, I would be more vulnerable to regaining the weight unless I created ways to switch off False Fixes with Healthy Fixes. I'm so grateful for this hard-won knowledge, and I've made it my life's mission to teach others how to control their False Fixes, shed the mental and physical weight, and free themselves to live the life they so much deserve.

What's Eating You?

From the moment when I split those jeans to right now, I've never regained those 50 pounds. When life gets me down—a broken ankle, extensive travel without a break—I've fluctuated a little bit in my weight with 5 pounds here, 10 pounds there. But I've managed to keep returning to my optimal weight precisely because I respect the power of False Fixes. I know what they're capable of. I know that when life is going nuts all around me, False Fixes are biding their time, just waiting to help "fix" my problems.

I reversed my initial weight gain. But I have permanent changes in my body. I grew many extra thousands of fat cells. They're still with me—they're just deflated. But their very presence means I will always be at higher risk of rapid regain, since the fat containers are there, waiting to be refilled.

Also, because I tasted the food-addicted waters, I can never reverse that memory. To this day, I can taste the bridge mix from 30-plus years ago. The difference is that the joy I derive from the mountain of Healthy Fixes I have accrued over time far outweighs any reward I *think* I might get from that bag of candy.

Because here's the deal: False Fixes also need *you* to be their accomplice. Have you ever said to yourself:

"I deserve this treat. I've been working hard."

"I'm just keeping it together as it is—I can't handle a diet right now."

"I'll never be as skinny as [Natalie Portman/Angelina Jolie/insert celebrity here], so why even bother?"

"It's *just* a [pizza, cookie, candy, cake, pie] anyway."

"Food is like a good friend. It's always there for me."

"It's too late for me—I'm too old to start trying to lose weight."

"What's the use? I always gain it back anyway."

Yes, you may be struggling with some food addiction. But if you've said any of these to yourself, watch out. You're also getting hooked on excuses, justifications, and rationalizations. You're enabling your own addiction.

You say you want to shed the weight and be able to run and dance and walk on the beach in a bathing suit again. Then why do you live in clutter and chaos, so that you can't find your sneakers, let alone schedule your gym time, because you're so disorganized?

Because *living that way* is also a False Fix. Maybe you are using your False Fix to numb the pain of: The abusive husband you fear leaving because you're scared of being on your own. The thankless, no-joy job you're too afraid to quit. The negative personality traits that push people away—your impatience, impulsivity, anger, or social withdrawal. Or the mother of all: The sense that you are not worthy, that you are bad, wrong, or unlovable. Too scared to change, you become hooked on the familiarity of it all. You'll live with the pain of your current life because somehow it's working for you. Like a child's beaten-up blankie you drag around with you, that familiar habit brings comfort—and that faux comfort is your reward.

You try to dissociate from your pain with many False Fixes. Food might only be one of them. Maybe you are also hooked on watching hours of reality TV. Or bidding on eBay for stuff you'll never use. Or stalking your ex on Facebook. Or Internet porn.

Maybe you like to gamble—a bit too much. Or gossip about your friends. Or troll Web sites, picking fights with faceless strangers. Or say yes to every request and remain ridiculously busy, so you never have to slow down and face the painful realities of your False Fix life.

All of these activities, every single one, taps into the hardwired

Am I a Food Addict?

Curious if you are under the spell of False Fix foods? Let's take a moment to see. The Yale Food Addiction Scale was developed by Yale research scientist Ashley Gearhardt and has been scientifically validated. This is a brief, user-friendly version to quickly assess whether you have a food addiction. (To take the full survey, see Appendix A.)

Instructions

Please answer the questions 1 through 7 using these numerical options:

0: Never

1: Once per month

2: 2 to 4 times per month

3: 2 to 3 times per week

4: 4+ times per week

1. I find myself consuming certain foods even though I am no longer hungry. _____

2. I worry about cutting down on certain foods. _____

3. I feel sluggish or fatigued from overeating. _____

4. I have spent time dealing with negative feelings from overeating certain foods, instead of spending time in important activities such as time with family, friends, work, or recreation. _____

5. I have had physical withdrawal symptoms such as agitation and anxiety when I cut down on certain foods. (Do NOT include caffeinated drinks: coffee, tea, cola, energy drinks, etc.) _____

reward system that's kept humans going since the beginning of existence. Not only do other mammals—rats, mice, apes—share the dopamine-linked brain reward circuitry, so do simple mollusks like slugs and snails. Even *amoebas*.[16] Some researchers believe dopamine was the catalyst for the development of intelligence. If we've been seeking out pleasure in the name of survival since we slithered out of the swamp,[17] you can be damn sure the reward system is powerful enough to trick you into eating an Oreo or watching *Jersey Shore*—even if your more cerebral side, your PFC, is totally mortified at the thought.

---

6. My behavior with respect to food and eating causes me significant distress. _____

7. Issues related to food and eating decrease my ability to function effectively (daily routine, job/school, social or family activities, health difficulties). _____

Then, answer Yes or No for questions 8 and 9.

8. I kept consuming the same types or amounts of food despite significant emotional and/or physical problems related to my eating. _____

9. Eating the same amount of food does not reduce negative emotions or increase pleasurable feelings the way it used to. _____

Scoring

To meet the food addiction criteria, you need to have answered "Yes" to either 8 or 9 (or both); AND met the scores below on three or more of the questions 1 through 7.

Question 1: 4	Question 4: 3 or 4	Question 7: 3 or 4
Question 2: 4	Question 5: 3 or 4	Question 8: Yes
Question 3: 3 or 4	Question 6: 3 or 4	Question 9: Yes

Now, before you throw your hands up in despair, I'm not saying that we can't outsmart our False Fixes. I did, and I know that you can, too. You want to reclaim your brain, your free will, and the ability to take control of your life. You *will* make this happen. The solution relies on exactly the same brain mechanisms that got us into this mess. Because, like it or not, we *will* be looking for our fixes for the rest of our lives—but we have the ability to choose *which* fixes.

The first step to freedom begins with acknowledging your dependence on False Fixes—this realization will also help you appreciate just how intoxicating your Healthy Fixes can be. In the next chapter, you'll learn about how the Hunger Fix cycle works—how it gets its early start, how it conditions and motivates us and influences our behavior, and how understanding and respecting the power of the cycle will actually set you free.

CHAPTER 2

The Hunger Fix Cycle

MAN IS NOT THE CREATURE OF CIRCUMSTANCES,
CIRCUMSTANCES ARE THE CREATURES OF MEN.
WE ARE FREE AGENTS, AND MAN
IS MORE POWERFUL THAN MATTER.
—BENJAMIN DISRAELI

EVERYTHING WE DO IN LIFE IS FOR A REWARD.
We have sex. Reward.
We laugh. Reward.
We fight. Reward.
We make up. Reward.

Learning, bonding, working, kissing—each and every action we do is automatically calculated to elicit the greatest reward. Our brain doesn't much care if those rewards come from snorting cocaine or running a marathon—it just wants that gold-star feeling.

To understand the power of reward, try this simple exercise. For one day, for every action you do—from hopping out of bed, to donning your cashmere sweater, to savoring your latte, to playing with your dog, to making that deadline at work and falling into bed at night—identify the reward associated with every action. Think of *where* you practiced each of these habits and how you felt about each: joyful, happy, satisfied, proud. Then consider: When you plow through a box of cookies, a family-size bag of chips, or five pieces of pizza, where are you now? Alone behind closed doors? How rewarded do you *feel*? If there's shame, guilt, and angst associated with that action, what was that reward again?

Whether your idea of a good time is a 3-mile hike at 6:00 a.m. or the three-scoop sundae at 6:00 p.m., you are getting a reward from that behavior. And the more you choose that particular reward, the more comfortable and accustomed to that reward your brain becomes, eventually resulting in a knee-jerk conditioned response: ice cream = reward. Your choice becomes a habit, nestled snugly in a well-worn path in your neuronal network.

Every False Fix in our lives started somewhere—sometimes before we were even born. What happens in our early lives can either protect us from these genetic predispositions or make us more vulnerable to these False Fix tendencies. Let's learn about where the hunger for those False Fixes begin, how it progresses, and how you can use all of this information to stop it in its tracks.

Fixed from the Start

When I said we'd looking at beginnings, I wasn't fooling around. Let's get molecular. The cells of your body contain *genes*, strings of the chemical DNA. Taken together, your entire collection of genes is referred to as the *genome*. The genome acts as a combination blueprint and instruction manual for your body, determining everything from what color your hair and eyes are to how each cell functions and what makes, say, a muscle cell different from a skin or liver cell.

You can think of the genome as a book, filled with genes that make up its sentences, paragraphs, and chapters. The pages of that book are filled with annotations. Some pages are bookmarked or dog-eared; others are stapled together and inaccessible. The annotations in your genetic book take the form of certain chemicals and molecules that attach themselves to the genes. Because they sit, in a sense, on top of the genome, this collection of annotations is called the *epi*genome, "epi" meaning above or outside.

Most cells in your body contain the entire genome; a cell in your heart contains not only the genes for a heart cell but also the genes for a liver cell, a nerve cell, a skin cell, and every other kind of cell. Yet that heart cell ignores all instructions that aren't heart-cell-related, the epigenome switching certain genes off and certain genes on.

All this switching is the work of special proteins called histones that surround each gene. Histones are genetic referees, scanning every action you take and choice you make, switching the message that particular gene will deliver to the rest of the body. Eat junk food and your genetic "speech" or expression changes, resulting in a whole cascade of biological changes, including increased body inflammatory processes. Eat an apple and histones order the gene to start a different cascade, resulting in improved immune function. Your job is to keep those histones scripting the healthiest messages possible. The goal is to have *happy histones* throughout your life.

Some genetic mutations will occur; it's the passing of those mutations to future generations that drives the process of evolution. But during your lifetime, you're pretty much stuck with the genes you're born with. What's exciting about the epigenome is that it adds new possibilities to that unchangeable genome, just as crossing out some paragraphs and emphasizing others could make a book like *Moby-Dick* seem like an entirely different story. Your DNA is not necessarily your destiny!

A striking example of this occurs in a breed of lab mouse called agouti. These mice have a certain gene—the agouti gene—that causes them to become obese and, as a unique molecular by-product of the activation of this obesity gene, also gives them yellow fur. The mice are also at high risk for developing heart disease, diabetes, and cancer. Yet scientists have observed that among agouti mice who have

exactly the same genes—which is to say, they are identical twins—
one mouse can develop yellow fur and obesity, while the other grows
up slim and with brown fur.

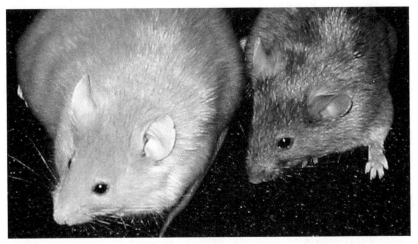

Genetically identical, these two mice show how great of an impact epigenetics can have.
The mother of the mouse on the left received a normal mouse diet; the mother of the mouse
on the right received a diet supplemented with methyl donors (choline, folic acid, betaine,
and vitamin B$_{12}$), which increased her baby's DNA methylation. (PHOTO © RANDY L. JIRTLE)

How is this possible, and why does it matter? The answer is epigenetics: In one mouse, that agouti gene has been switched off, and so
the yellow fur and obesity don't develop. In this case, the gene is
marked "do not read" because a specific molecule, called a methyl
group, has been attached to it. The process is called *methylation*. As
it turns out, dietary interventions kept the agouti gene from being
activated. Researchers simply supplemented the obese yellow mother's diet with methyl donors like vitamin B$_{12}$, choline, betaine, and
folic acid or genistein, a phytoestrogen food in soy products. The
mouse pups were born with brown fur, lean and at no risk for disease. This was a groundbreaking experiment and officially established the food-gene connection, as well as helped mark the birth of
the science of epigenetics. This methylation is an important way that
the epigenome exerts its effects, not just in mice but in us, too.

The agouti mice give us another example of prenatal epigenetics at work. When pregnant mice were given a chemical called BPA— bisphenol A, an additive found in plastics, which is known to suppress methylation (and thus keep the obesity gene turned on)—their offspring developed the yellow fur and obesity that are the hallmarks of their breed. But in a group of mice who were fed a diet that supports methylation (the human equivalent of eating more broccoli, asparagus, eggs, peas, vegetarian baked beans, salmon, and rainbow trout), the offspring tended to be slim and brown. (Lends new meaning to "You are what you eat"!)

Let's look at how epigenetics works with food addiction. A diet full of unhealthy fat, salt, sugar, and processed-food chemicals switches on certain genes to cope with it. Savoring too much refined and processed sugar? Those histones get busy directing the genes to increase insulin secretion. This starts a domino effect that includes the stimulation of fat storage, and with chronic exposure to sugar, insulin resistance occurs and type 2 diabetes can result. Eating too much food in general? The body adapts to maintain survival. Out comes the genetic message to create more fat cells to store the excess fuel. Those excess fat cells then create higher levels of leptin, a hormone secreted near the fat cells that communicates fat storage status to the brain. This excess fat also increases the level of inflammation in the body, activating other genes that result in more pain in body parts vulnerable to inflammatory influences, such as your joints (arthritis) or your gut (colitis).

If the overeating continues on a chronic basis, the body eventually adapts and these foods become the body's new normal. And, based on the brain changes and newly hijacked reward system, the body begins to crave these foods. You hunger for them. You're addicted; your False Fixes are fully engaged.

Epigenetic changes can last through several generations. Swedish researchers have found higher mortality rates in people whose grandparents lived through a famine. And a study of US children whose mothers had gastric bypass surgery found that kids were much less likely to be obese if they were born after the surgery than before (when the mother was still overweight and overeating). In both cases, epigenetic inheritance is the likely explanation: Certain genes were switched on or off in both moms and dads, and the instructions for those genes to be active or not were inherited by their descendants.

We're only beginning to understand how epigenetics works and what it means for human health. But recent research suggests that the subject is a bigger game changer than we thought. You may not be able to change your genes, but you have a powerful role to play in helping to direct how those genes communicate and collaborate with the rest of the mind and body. And that self-directed genetic speech writing can be lifesaving. Whatever you do in your life, from sitting too much to running 3 miles every day, those histones are making nanosecond-by-nanosecond adjustments to keep you alive. If you can change certain key choices—your diet, the way you handle stress, how you move your body—you can rewrite those notes in the margins of your genome and flip the switch to activate the genes that support and protect your health. As the genes underlying that addiction are turned on, your False Fix cravings will decrease enough for you to be able to control your choices and shed the weight.

Yes, addiction does create a permanent memory in your genome. Once you've tasted the addictive waters, your hormones, your brain, even your genes never forget. That's why you have to remain vigilant. Consistent healthy lifestyle choices have a very powerful impact on dampening the permanent effects enough to shed the weight as well as the disease risks. When those histones are happy at the epigenome, we reap those benefits. The choices are ours to make. Fat yellow mouse or slim brown mouse? It's up to us—and I'll show you how.

Now let's take a look at all the factors that may have tipped your genetic and epigenetic balance toward an addiction to False Fixes. Keep your own story in mind as you read, so you can spot your potential weaknesses. (We'll use that information in Chapter 4 to help you develop your own personal Healthy Fix plan.)

ADDICTIVE GENES

Among some of us, False Fixes start even before birth. Studies have found as much as 40 to 60 percent of our vulnerability to addiction can be directly linked to our genes—and 70 percent of the variability in our body mass index can as well.[1] People who have addictive genes—specifically carriers of A1 allele of the ANKK1 Taq1A polymorphism—will naturally have a shortage of the dopamine receptor known as D2. These are the receptors that can get wiped out from the continuous dopamine flooding—so people who are carriers of this polymorphism are already at a disadvantage, even before a bite of food comes to their lips. Double or triple this effect if you have more than one addiction. These cross-addictions hammer the reward system and seriously deplete your precious dopamine receptors. (Don't worry. I'll teach you a way around this common challenge.)

PRE- AND POSTNATAL DIET

Epigenetics is not solely a maternal issue. Although most of the research has been done on women, recent studies now show that dad's lifestyle choices and epigenetic changes are also transferred to his offspring. So, heads-up to *both* men and women thinking about starting a family. This is a terrific incentive to clean up your act not just for yourselves but to gift your future children with a chance to live a healthier life.

Fetuses in the womb drink several ounces of amniotic fluid every day. The developing baby can taste the specific flavors of whatever mom eats or drinks—and will show a preference for them after birth.[2] If Mom eats a lot of high-fat, high-sugar foods, the fetal reward system will develop an affinity for them as well.[3] Junk-food moms produce junk-food babies.

Mom's prenatal diet doesn't just impact her baby's taste buds or risk of obesity later in life—it can even set the child up for deadly diseases. Research funded by the British Heart Foundation says that poor maternal diet can cause epigenetic changes that reduce the expression of the gene Hnf4a, which has been linked to diabetes. Later in life, this epigenetic change can decrease the ability of the pancreas to make insulin, thereby raising the risk of type 2 diabetes.[4]

Finally, once a baby is born, any exposure to sweet tastes offers an early taste for our oldest natural reward[5] and one of the most common lifelong False Fixes: sugar.

EARLY EXPOSURE TO SUGAR

Sugar has such a strong effect on our brain chemistry that it has been used as an anesthetic during dental procedures and circumcision for small children. But doctors have noted that this painkilling effect stops working very quickly, and children outgrow it after just a few applications. Just like an adult who needs more and more Advil to kill headache pain, kids quickly develop a "tolerance" to sugar.

A study published in the journal *Addiction* found that children from families with addictive backgrounds outgrow this pain relief effect much sooner than kids from "normal" families, and they also show a strong preference for higher concentration of sweetness.[6] This preference is yet more evidence of a genetic vulnerability to cross-addiction of several different substances of abuse.

Now, bearing this vulnerable predisposition in mind, take a quick second to reflect on all the sugar that entered your life as a small child:

Lollipops at the bank.

Cake and ice cream and candy at birthday parties.

A cookie to make the knee scrape feel better.

Valentine's Day.

Easter baskets.

Hanukkah gelt.

Halloween.

And those are just the obvious ones. Even that small bowl of virtuous-sounding Honey Nut Cheerios in the morning had more sugar than three chocolate chip cookies.[7] Simple everyday applications of sugar increased the threshold of tolerance dramatically at a very young age.

In the first 3 years of life, our brains develop faster than at any other point in our lives. Those histones surrounding our epigenome are scanning what's being consumed and changing up the gene's message to the rest of our body. So if we feed children with processed foods, we're setting them up for increased addiction and disease risks.

Some of this is permanent. One study found that when 3-year-olds ate a high-fat/high-sugar diet of predominantly processed foods, their IQs were lower at age 8—regardless of whether their diet had improved in the interim.[8] Another study found half of children whose BMI was termed "high-rising" at age 2½ were obese by 8.[9]

Now, please don't think I'm some kind of party pooper. I'm not! I simply want to help you understand how much your reward system has been hammered with sugar from birth through adulthood. What I'm describing is the potential enormity of exposure to sugar from a variety of sources in our daily diet, some obvious and some quite subtle. (Ketchup has 4 grams per *teaspoon*—and we've all seen how kids seem to slurp up gallons of the stuff!) "Like kids in a candy store," we unconsciously upped our tolerance for sugar way before we knew of the long-term effects. Even if we didn't have the addictive gene, our environment was priming our DNA to change and *become* addictive. Heaven help you if you have the addictive gene *and* your environment was feeding you mountains of sweet crack!

PARENTAL LOVE

Several other factors can mix with your genetic tendencies during this very vulnerable time, things that have nothing to do with food. Babies who are held more, stroked more, sung to, and breastfed all develop lower stress reactivity. Their entire nervous systems are mellowed out—

which may help them resist addiction later on. Researchers believe one factor at play is a molecule in the brain's immune system called interleukin-10, which helps to decrease the reward effect that drugs such as morphine have in the brain. One Australian study on rats shows that pups who were stroked and nurtured by their mothers produced four times more IL-10 than control rats. When later exposed to the morphine, the pups didn't get addicted—and this mama-love protection created happy histones and thus positive epigenetic changes that persisted into adulthood, shielding the pups from morphine addiction for life.[10]

EARLY NEGLECT OR TRAUMA

On the other hand, if our early life is tumultuous or feels unsafe, it can leave us stripped and vulnerable to stress and addiction. If we suffer a trauma—either losing or being separated from a parent, or sexual or emotional abuse, or other traumatic experiences—our bodies develop

Protect Your Kids

Okay, so your parents didn't know. They poured the Cap'n Crunch and thought they were giving you a treat—not potentially dooming you to addiction. So how can you help your kids maximize their epigenetics and hopefully lower their chances of food addiction? A poll conducted by the University of Sydney found that certain parental habits could either protect kids from obesity or increase their risk.[11]

False Fix Habits	Healthy Fix Habits
Serve fast food for meals.	Serve water at meals.
Allow TV in kid's room.	Create rules about TV watching.
Have soda sitting around.	Limit intake of soda.
Take short car trips instead of walking or biking.	Encourage kids to be active.
Eat dinner in front of the TV.	Serve healthy breakfast every day.

a heightened sensitivity to stress. We might develop negative beliefs about ourselves and the world ("I'll never amount to anything"; "No one is ever going to love me"), and those beliefs can be retriggered whenever we encounter tough times—which can drive us headlong into the bar, the smoking lounge, another abusive relationship, or the refrigerator. Men who've endured trauma tend to act out, with aggression, violence, and rages. Women tend to turn inward, experiencing more anxiety, isolation, and depression. They may begin to *dissociate*, a term that means to mentally and physically disconnect from yourself and your identity. As a result, both men and women can start to use self-destructive habits—cutting, substance abuse, overeating—in a desperate attempt to cope with their angst and pain.

Among adult women who are addicts, 74 percent report sexual abuse, 52 percent report physical abuse, and 72 percent report emotional abuse.[12] Among women who binge eat, 83 percent were abused as children. Often when addicts "fall off the wagon" or have trouble with their recovery, it is because they're still struggling to deal with their earlier traumas—and they revert to self-medicating with their False Fix.

EARLY STRESS

Another thing that stress does is directly impact our prefrontal cortex. You recall that the PFC is the most highly evolved part of our brain, one that helps us resist temptation, reins in impulses, keeps us organized, and directs our mind to long-term goals. Studies have shown that social stress impairs our ability to maintain attention and disrupts communication between several parts of our brain.[13] Even a brief burst of stress can cause a rapid and dramatic loss of our PFC's ability to think. If that stress goes on much longer, it can start to cause architectural changes in the prefrontal dendrites, the branches that reach off of our neurons to communicate with other brain cells.[14] The PFC is our strongest ally in the fight against False Fixes—but unfortunately, it is also the brain region most sensitive to stress.

ATTENTION DEFICIT HYPERACTIVITY DISORDER

Impulsivity is a hallmark of ADHD and of addiction. And no wonder the two have so much in common: People who have the highest impulsivity scores have the lowest activity in their midbrain D2/D3 dopamine receptors, the same receptors that have been linked with food addiction.[15] If you were a child with undiagnosed (or untreated) ADHD, you are two to three times more likely to develop substance abuse problems.[16] (Self-medicating, anyone?) One study found that one in three women who had childhood ADHD later became food addicts.[17]

TEENAGE DRUG ABUSE

Because the PFC is not fully developed until we are 25, we see plenty of bad decision making during the teen years. Peppered with their volatile mix of hormones, teens' growing brains are drawn to high-thrill/low-demand activities—in other words, they are sitting ducks for False Fixes. Sadly, any teenage alcohol and drug experimentation can take a tremendous long-term toll. Chronic drinking during the teen years causes significant brain damage in the frontal cortex and massive neuron loss in the hippocampus, a memory center, shrinking it by upward of 10 percent. Cigarette smoking is often the gateway drug to drinking and harder drugs, because it so quickly and efficiently whets the appetite for False Fixes. Ten seconds after your very first drag on a cigarette, nicotine releases dopamine and drenches half of your reward system's acetylcholine receptors—and, by the end of the cigarette, almost all of the receptors have been touched. The brain shows signs of addiction to nicotine after just three cigarettes— far before a peer-pressured teen even begins to consciously enjoy lighting up. Nicotine also suppresses MAO, an enzyme that "cleans up" excess dopamine in the brain.[18] With less MAO, the dopamine flooding cycle begins—priming the pump for all other addictions, including food. In fact, at this age, teens may even start consciously abusing food as a drug, as captured in one teen's post online:

It's like a drug. What used to satisfy you before now has no effect. I feel like I've become immune to foods that used to comfort me. And like drugs, you keep moving on to bigger, worse things in order to get the same feeling as when you started out.[19]

At 14, this girl was 5 feet 2 and weighed 201 pounds.

Stacking the Odds

Flash forward several decades. Now, as adults, we live with the combined effects of all of those earlier life experiences. We might celebrate with food or use it to self-medicate or both. We try to stop. But we feel powerless to stop. And in today's toxic food environment, it's really no wonder why.

Lab rats will quickly develop a tolerance for sugar, eagerly *quadrupling* their daily sugar consumption in 1 week. If the sugar's taken away, the hunger for their fix is relentless and they'll go through withdrawal—start fighting with the other rats, shaking, getting angry. And once they've become addicted to sugar, they are far more eager to gobble up amphetamines, alcohol, and cocaine in huge quantities, and they become almost instantly addicted to those as well. But when given the choice between sugar, cocaine, and alcohol, those cross-addicted rats will always choose—you guessed it—the sugar.[20]

Substance abuse researchers say that the brain adaptations that result from regularly eating so-called hyperpalatable foods—foods that layer salt, fat, and sweet flavors, proven to increase consumption—are likely to be more difficult to change than those from cocaine or alcohol because they involve many more neural pathways. Almost 90 percent of the dopamine neurons in the ventral tegmental area (VTA) of the brain are activated in response to food cues.[21] In an fMRI study, among women who tested higher for food addiction, just thinking about drinking a chocolate milk shake stimulated greater activation in the anterior cingulate cortex, medial orbitofrontal cortex, and amygdala, all brain areas involved in emotion, anticipation, and decision making. And rats who received highly palatable food for only 2 weeks showed a decrease in gene expression for enkephalin, a natural painkiller, in the nucleus accumbens—the same changes found in brain chemistry of chronic morphine or heroin addicts.[22]

Brand-new research also shows direct evidence of lasting and fundamental injuries to a part of the brain that helps us regulate our food intake, the hypothalamic arcuate nucleus. Within 3 days of being placed on a high-fat diet, a rat's hypothalamus shows increased inflammation; within a week, researchers see evidence of permanent scarring and neuron injury in an area of the brain crucial for weight control.

I Need a Fix

The Siren Call of the Visual Cue

Read Bonnie's description of the magnetic attraction of the cues from her personal False Fix crack den, the fast-food joint:

> Last week I received a McDonald's coupon book in the mail. And I swear that I could smell french fries as soon as I saw it. Just a McDonald's commercial on TV or a McDonald's "drive by" triggers that smell in my head.
>
> All of my senses are triggered at the sight or mere knowledge and vicinity of a fast-food location that sells all of the items that are filled with grease and that used to bring me calm in a world of crazy. When I did not have someone to talk to, I could comfort myself with a bag full of greasy comfort. Now it seems really odd. While I crave and want the KFC or Popeyes, I have to ask myself if it is truly worth the physical cost or would I rather take care of myself in a healthier way. Lately, the answer has been, "Go work out—I will get the same feeling of satisfaction."

Brain scans on obese men and women show this exact pattern as well.[23]

Add in all the hormonal changes, your emotional connections to food, peer pressure, 3:00 p.m. grogginess, deadline stress, and your body's drive to feed your new fat cells. Finally, consider that the longer you've been consuming your favorite False Fix (since your first birthday cupcake, perhaps?), the more deeply entrenched all of those automatic responses have become.

Just look at how many different ways we strengthen the associations of a False Fix simultaneously with one fast-food meal:

On a habitual level . . . by mindlessly driving past the same burger joint during the same hungry commuting time, every single day—seeing the brightly colored sign, smelling the burger grease, remembering the "great deal" coupons you have in your glove box—all cues that have been linked together and hardwired on instructions from the prefrontal cortex.

On an emotional level . . . by telling ourselves, during stressful times or when we're tired or lonely, that we "deserve a treat," thinking that cheeseburger is a "friend" who can soothe away a fight with a loved one or a disheartening day at the office.

On a neurochemical level . . . by ingesting a meal consciously designed in preparation, ingredients, and portion size to manipulate our brain chemistry, with additives and nutrients that release that familiar dopamine rush as well as an opium-like rush of pleasure that also becomes addictive. (Mom had Valium, Dad had scotch and cigarettes, we have . . . a Dairy Queen Large Chocolate Chip Cookie Dough Blizzard?)

On a hormonal level . . . by overtaxing our insulin, ghrelin, and leptin hunger/satiety systems with toxic trans fats, copious corn syrup, and extra calories until they are "resistant," no longer able to balance our blood sugar or respond with natural fullness cues—causing us to eat even more.

On a cellular level . . . by adding extra fat cells to our bodies that, once born, can never be removed and, instead, through decreased leptin levels, trigger ever-stronger appetite signals.

On a *genetic* **level . . .** by reacting to overeating of hyperpalatable foods and changing our genes' expression within as little time as 2 weeks—which serves only to reinforce the entire cycle over and over and over again.[24]

Addiction research shows that abusing drugs leads to changes in the way we perceive emotions, make decisions, remember things— even slowing our motor reflexes.[25] When our False Fix is food addiction, changes like these not only hijack our normal motivations and signals to eat but also damage our body's ability to burn off the food efficiently by changing our metabolic set point.

Which all ends up with one outcome: We become fatter and more addicted.

Give Yourself Some Credit

I hope you're starting to understand why the message "eat less, move more" as the solution for weight management is just not going to cut it anymore. And why telling overweight and obese people to "just pull it together, get some willpower, and stop eating so much" is way out of sync with the new science of food addiction—not to mention frustrating and even hurtful to those who suffer from it. The reality is, if you are food addicted, you have been dealt a uniquely challenging hand. I'm as resentful as you are when folks throw volleys of platitudes like "It's so simple—calories in, calories out!" Instead of being stigmatized, struggling food addicts deserve the highest respect and support.

Just think of what it takes a junkie to get off heroin in rehab:

The junkie is locked up in a guarded facility, safe from all temptation, and given an opportunity to go "cold turkey" with every possible physical, mental, and emotional support. He doesn't have to go to work; he has no immediate family stress.

In this bubble, he is coached through hours and hours of intensive group and individual therapy (possibly even given a pharmaceutical drug to reduce cravings). The junkie is then greeted by delighted family members who cry with gratitude and pride that he's made it this far, and linked up with a mentor for help after he's released.

Once he's out, he has regularly scheduled meetings with supportive fellow junkies who congratulate him for not having shot up for another month, week, or even day. Everyone around him acknowledges how every single day is a struggle for him. They say things like "I'm so proud of you—you are so strong."

Recovering heroin addicts have all this help, and yet 87 percent of junkies coming out of rehab will *still* relapse.

Now consider this: If you are addicted to food, you *are* that junkie. And you've been locked in a drug den with limitless supplies of dope—no going cold turkey from food!—with constant pressure from relentless deadlines and chores and social pressures.

The food junkie has to sit through commercials on TV that say, "What are you waiting for—you remember! Shooting up is simply amazing! Everyone else is doing it! Go on—you *deserve* it!"

The food junkie has friends standing around, shoving full syringes at her, saying, "This stuff is absolutely the best—just try it! C'mon, a little taste . . . "

Your mom is even there, looking wounded, saying, "What do you mean, you don't want to try my heroin? I made it just for you!"

And all you want to say is *"Doesn't anyone understand the hell I'm going through?"*

I do. I understand you and your struggle. Give yourself a tremendous amount of credit. You are about to take on one of your greatest challenges—overcoming food addiction—and, with *The Hunger Fix*, you're going to knock it out of the park. Let's see how the three-stage path to freedom works!

CHAPTER 3

Breaking the Hunger Fix Cycle

YOU WANT TO SEE A MIRACLE, SON? BE THE MIRACLE.
—GOD COACHING BRUCE, *BRUCE ALMIGHTY*

W HEN FALSE FIXES HAVE SO MANY TENTACLES with which to control us, how can we possibly defend ourselves against them?

Answer: We get high the *right* way, and we stay that way.

We know these motivation-learning-memory reward circuits are hardwired into us on a molecular level. There's no way we're going to evolve out of them. The reward process itself is never going to change, nor should it. Our only option is get the science on our side, to learn to tap into our own reward system and make it work *for* us instead of against us.

In this chapter, we'll look at how the Hunger Fix program works, retraining the reward system to prefer natural, pleasurable, sustainable, life-enhancing Healthy Fixes instead of the seductive lies of the False Fixes that promise immediate ecstasy but end up leaving us filled with guilt and self-loathing. The key to success is being able to prefer, and therefore choose, one reward over another. I'll also explain the progression of each stage of the plan—why *these* steps work in *this* order to grow the brain while shrinking the waistline. Your new mantra is "Big Brain, Small Waist." The entire Hunger Fix plan works with your brain to maximize your changing neurochemistry at each stage of this three-stage progression, with the critical elements augmenting each other as you go.

The Dopamine System Can Rebuild Itself

Your brain is capable of a broad range of reward responses. Our job is to help you fine-tune your brain and find that optimal and satisfying level of pleasure, derived from your own *natural* reward system. Reward is primal and has been in existence in all creatures in evolutionary history. But we humans differ from the amoeba and the snail in that our mammalian reward system is complex—it intersects with our executive functions, emotions, memories, dreams, and aspirations, all of which reside in different areas of our brain.

The dopamine in our brain is actually dispersed in many different areas. At the start of the Hunger Fix program, we focus on one particular area—the ventral tegmental area (VTA), in which almost 90 percent of the dopamine neurons get stimulated when we're about to eat. The VTA reaches out to the rest of the brain via many axons (long fingerlike extensions from neurons) to transmit electrical impulses that stimulate dopamine secretion in several different areas, including the mesolimbic and mesocortical dopamine systems. The mesolimbic system reaches into the nucleus accumbens (the site of reward, pleasure, and addiction), the amygdala (where emotions are processed and remembered), and the hippocampus (a site that converts short-term to long-term memory).[1]

When dopamine is released into the space between the neurons, it starts to do its work by binding with dopamine receptors. The dopamine in those receptors then communicates messages of pleasure to other parts of the brain and then undergoes reuptake and recycling for use later somewhere else. Cocaine and amphetamines cause a dopamine "rush" because they allow the dopamine to linger in this space between neurons and to activate the dopamine receptors even longer, resulting in a more intense high. Yet brain scan studies and blood tests suggest sugar and other sweet tastes even surpass this drug high.[2]

Any kind of fix that activates dopamine-containing neurons of the VTA and releases dopamine into any of those target brain areas will be felt as pleasurable. And, like Pavlov's dogs, we have very long, strong memories of pleasure that get stored in many parts of the brain. Once we've tasted the waters of pleasure and reward, we'll remember them forever. We may not salivate at the sound of a bell, but all of the sights, sounds, smells, or thoughts—any sensory cue or action—that preceded and overlapped those pleasurable experiences will then be associated with those positive feelings. Every time we repeat those experiences, those associations get more intense and those neural pathways get stronger—and following each rush, we use our PFC to help us figure out how to get the next "hit." For example, fat is extremely palatable for the very purpose of survival. One taste is all it took to convince primitive people to put out the effort to seek and eat it at every opportunity. And thank heavens for that, since Paleolithic communities needed fat fuel to endure the frequent famines. Our innate fat preference is just another example of Mother Nature watching our backs.

From our first ice-cream cone to the sight of a crimson sunset to that first kiss, our PFC assigns a "price tag" based on the initial experience: How much effort do I need to put out to repeat this again . . . and again? We could get this same benefit from a hot date—or a gallon of Ben & Jerry's. We could get it from a platter of nachos—

or from meditation, prayer, volunteering, exercise, a feeling of community, affirmations from others. We can get a sense of immediate pleasure from either end of the spectrum—but it's the PFC making the decision as to which one is actually "worth it."

For many of us, that's a tough choice. The gray matter in our PFC, the actual nerve cells that help us make decisions and retain self-control, have been damaged to the point where we can no longer remember the long-term, more authentic benefits of the runner's high or the helper's high—we can only remember the superquick high we get when we dive into a double cheeseburger, warm buttered bread, or a thickly iced double-chocolate birthday cake.[3] We've tipped over into delay discounting: The pain now is simply not worth the pleasure later. We'll take the hamburger today, sir.

My friend and colleague, former FDA commissioner David Kessler, MD, wrote *The End of Overeating.* Having waged his own battles with obesity, Dr. Kessler recounted a particular struggle with a False Fix of his.

> I walked into a bakery in San Francisco and asked for two semi-sweet chocolate chip cookies. Back home, I pulled the cookies out of their bag and placed them on a paper plate, just beyond my arm's reach. They were thick and gooey—chunks of chocolate filled the craters of the cookies and rose into peaks.
>
> I focused my attention on them, monitoring my own response. I sighed deeply and bit my lower lip. Almost indifferent to the flowers on the table and even to the framed photos of my children on the counter, I was fixated on those cookies until I forced myself to pull away. At some point I noticed that I had moved my right hand a few inches closer to them, but I had no conscious recollection of my decision to

act. I tried to concentrate on reading the newspaper, but I kept glancing back to the plate.

Feeling vaguely uneasy, I headed to my upstairs office, which is about as far away from the kitchen as I can get. But even from that safe distance, I could not fully shake the image of the cookies. Eventually, I left the house without having eaten them, and I felt triumphant.

Hours later, I headed to Café Greco where the cappuccino is said to be the best in the city. A large glass jar filled with homemade cookies sat on the counter.

I ordered an orange-chocolate cookie and ate it at once.

We see delay discounting in rat experiments—they'll ignore their babies, stop eating, do nothing but press a lever up to 7,000 times an hour to deliver a "high" to their reward centers. They'll quickly turn into coke addicts, continuing to hit the lever over and over in order to get the cocaine-laced food.

But one thing separates us from those rats: our PFC. That most sensitive and evolved part of our brains is the link between what excites our reward centers and our ultimate goals. The PFC helps us see beyond the usual "vices" like fatty goods, sugar, sex, etc. to the more meaningful rewards, the Healthy Fixes that feel good now *and* keep us mentally and physically strong long-term.

Strengthening the PFC, and thus reclaiming our hijacked reward system, is the "how" of the Hunger Fix program. By helping the PFC function better, we train it to choose the Healthy Fix—the choice that both immediately increases the amount of dopamine available throughout the brain *and* protects the reward system and optimizes our lifesaving genetic expression in the long-term. So by the time you're running your first 5-K, all of the memories and experiences—

from the sights, smells, and sweat to the hyperfocus, vigilance, and fortitude to the blissful exhilaration at finishing—will be wrapped into one big package of pleasure in the end.

Reveal Your Real Hunger

This whole motivation-learning-memory-reward circuit interplay has not escaped the attention of legal as well as illegal enterprises looking to capitalize on the weakness of vulnerable and susceptible people with addictive tendencies. Be it providing porn, cigarettes, shopping, gambling, online trades, illegal drugs, or processed foods, these folks want to walk away with your reward system and generate income while they're at it. At the same time, we have an entire diet industry that points the finger at the consumer and says, "You just have to learn— here are some fat gram charts and a pair of sneakers. Now, go knock yourselves out." As renowned Canadian obesity researcher Arya Sharma, MD, says, expecting an addicted person to kick the overeating habit by simply reading a food label is like expecting a crack addict to go clean after attending a lecture on the dangers of crack addiction.

The fact that you keep expecting yourself to change on your own— and blaming yourself when you cannot—just feeds the problem. You feel like a failure and sink further into your retreat, your dissociation. It can make some people feel like pariahs in their own culture—yet when they try to fight their way out, they're labeled as failures there, too. Better to simply not try.

When I see an announcement about a study on food addiction, I feel encouraged—the science is finally catching up with what my patients have wrestled with for years. But then the op-ed pages and the airwaves and the message boards fill up with the inevitable backlash— "just stop eating, fatties!"—and, I have to admit, it drives me crazy. When are we going to wake up?

If we can all acknowledge how incredibly hard this is—because it's a conscious business decision to make it hard *to eat just one*—then we can have a compassionate discussion about how to get clean from False Fixes. We can start to tap into that elegant reward circuitry to do the things that will truly benefit us, things that bring health and life and vitality and passion and no more guilt or shame or pain.

I know you are hurting. I know you've been down this road so many times. But you *can* do this. You *can* transform your false hunger into an authentic, healthy hunger that will fuel you to Detox from your False Fixes and help you transition into a joyful and rewarding lifelong recovery. My patients and I are living proof that you can recapture your life and break free from these False Fixes that want to own your brain. They can't own it unless you let them.

Florence Griffith Joyner, the former American Olympic gold medalist in the sprint and fastest woman in the world, was once asked to share her secrets of success. She said, "Three words: believe, achieve, succeed." Many have repeated this since, and I concur wholeheartedly. Freedom begins with a belief that you can kick your False Fixes and regain control of your life. The brain will follow whatever you believe. You'll strengthen your PFC, which leads to enlightenment, mindfulness, and better choices—a jog is better for me, feels more satisfying than sitting on a couch, eating a huge bowl of ice cream. That's why the Hunger Fix begins with a powerful driver to get you through Detox. The only thing that's going to break you free is this: You have to *want it, really bad*.

You have to dig deep, past the False Hunger that's trying to trick you, to the Real Hunger—what is it that's going to help you resist the urge to reach back into the candy bag or to sneak down to the 7-Eleven for a tube of Pringles at 1 o'clock in the morning? You have to have a purpose so true, a hunger so strong, that any piddling little craving you have is going to have a bitch of a time fighting you for that dopamine receptor.

FIRST, FIND YOUR EpiphaME

You need an epiphany. An Epipha*ME*. Something must happen to create a perceivable "click" deep inside your mind. Suddenly you get it. Within a nanosecond, the reward system does a 180 and you're headed for significant change in your life.

Someone says that unless you drop weight, you'll be on insulin. Boom. Game over.

You meet the love of your life who's in great shape and you're not. You want to share biking and running and fun outdoors with him. Then your pants rip while you're on a hike together. Boom. You're in the gym and workin' it.

You're in the ER with chest pain and shortness of breath, terrified and splayed out on a gurney. Got your attention now?

Or you're just sick and tired of feeling sick and tired and overweight. Not even your fail-safe False Fixes work anymore. You see them for what they are—the drug that sucks the life out of you, leaving you to shy away from social events and to withdraw from the joys of life you dream about as you fall asleep in yet another food coma.

You've hit rock bottom. And this makes one hell of an EpiphaME to power the launch of your Healthy Fix journey.

You always know when your EpiphaME has occurred because your BMW (bitch, moan, whine) all but disappears. Your attitude starts to change from "Man, it's such a pain to go to the gym and I feel too tired and it's too cold to drive there, and my workout buddy can't make it so I'm not going" to "Man, I wish that guy would get the hell off the elliptical already since I need to use it!!" and "Rain? No problem, I'll pop on my raincoat and walk anyway."

To get a sense of where you stand right now, for the next 24 hours write down any excuse that pours from your lips as you make self-care choices. From deciding whether to meditate or journal or grocery shop or take that walk, be very aware of your decision making. When your PFC is fully engaged, the BMW chatter is almost nil.

When that excuse maker is gone, you're home. That dopamine receptor is yours—you own it. You're going to stimulate it to produce a tsunami of pleasure with Healthy Fix foods that feed your soul, not your addictive beast. You're going to feel the joy and reward from the physical movement and exercise that flood your body with dopamine, that help regrow your receptors instead of destroy them.

Let's create your EpiphaME—you and me, together. To prepare you for the Hunger Fix program, in Chapter 4 I will lead you through a process to uncover your Healthy Hunger, the reason you have buried deep in your PFC, the motivating force that will drive you through the valley of bottomless chips, cookies, and french fries and back to a younger, happier, fitter, more exhilarated you. We'll figure out where your problems began so we can map the best path possible. We'll toss out all the old crap that's sitting in your house just waiting to drag you back in. We are going to win back your brain from those False Fixes—the beast be damned!

Once you have your EpiphaME, you're ready for the Hunger Fix.

Stage 1: False Fix Detox: Getting Your Natural Dopamine High

This is a kinder, gentler Detox.

I'll help you make the switch from False to Healthy Fixes and, by doing so, begin rebuilding your motivation-learning-memory reward circuits to support your new "habit." There's no staring at a pile of bean sprouts for dinner. Deprivation leads to stress, which leads to stress eating. Instead, you'll enjoy tasty, delicious, and satisfying foods.

In a traditional detox, when the addict suddenly stops "using," dopamine receptors can return to the original levels—but it takes some time. That transition time is typically characterized by withdrawal—anxiety, agitation, irritability, impatience, headaches, a feeling of unease. It can be mentally and physically uncomfortable, even painful. And, science is finding, probably even counterproductive.

As brutal as traditional drug abuse recovery was, it was also very simple: You get off your drug, and changes start happening immediately— it's just one substance. (Unless, of course, you are addicted.) Food is unfortunately more complex. First of all, you have to eat to survive. Second, most people are addicted to combinations of flavors—savory, salty, starchy; or sweet and fat; or fat and starchy. Therefore, it takes longer for the adaptation process to take place. And that's before you bring in all the other issues—conditioned response, cultural expectations, depression, stress eating. Your mom.

The Hunger Fix Detox avoids the traditional brutal deprivation period. Why? Science has shown that when you eliminate all False Fixes and leave that person with nothing that can adequately match and substitute for the False Fix high, you create lots of stress. Cortisol levels rise, exacerbating your chemical withdrawal, stimulating a stress-induced appetite—and there you are, back to bingeing voraciously on your False Fix foods.

The Hunger Fix Detox gives you a soft landing into your post-food-addiction life. In Stage 1, I'm particularly interested in the dopamine activity in the mesolimbic part of the system—it has a greater role in emotional expression, motivation, and reward. So you'll first work on getting that area of the brain soothed and on an even keel. Instead of gutting it out over the din of a growling stomach and a pile of celery sticks, you will fill your belly with Healthy Fix foods and distract your brain with a lot of sustainable, healthy, dopamine-boosting rewards to draw on—cooking classes, physical activity, decluttering, making new friends, taking on new projects—so it never has time to miss your False Fixes. You'll be stimulating neurogenesis and increasing the number of dopamine receptors while you begin to engage and beef up your PFC. The simple act of saying no to False Fixes and saying yes to Healthy Fixes is like a push-up for your PFC.

Then, when you experience the dopamine rush from your Healthy Fix, you'll further reinforce the experience in your PFC, which will make the next no that much easier—and the next and the next. This transfer from False to Healthy Fixes means that your brain is beginning to learn and accept that the reward from the Healthy Fix is now greater than the reward from the False Fix. This is the process of adaptation—your brain is making changes that ultimately could reroute your entire life.

During Detox, you do have to be patient. It takes a while to start rebuilding your dopamine receptors. After 40 days on a junk-food diet, fat-feasting rats will go on a hunger strike and refuse to eat any regular chow for 2 weeks.[4] They're holding out for their False Fix high, almost starving themselves to death! But somewhere around the 2-week mark, they start crawling back to the healthy food. Not coincidentally, this is exactly the same amount of time it takes for them to regain their lost dopamine receptors.[5]

While we can't know for sure how long it will take you to regain your lost receptors, most of the basic biological withdrawal—if you have any—should be resolved in about 3 or 4 weeks. Had those rat experiments continued, I'm sure we'd have seen them get more and more adapted to the normal chow and happily eat it every day—at which point, they'd be going from Rat Detox to Rat Beginner Recovery.

The key in Detox is to remember: The risk of relapse is high. You need to clean up the persons, places, and things in your life that provide the cues that trigger your food addiction, not just because it will make your life less stressful. The real reason is because your brain makes decisions about 10 seconds before you are consciously aware of them.[6] Your brain is actually more addicted to the *anticipation* of the False Fixes than to the fixes themselves. The fewer cues to remind us, the less deprivation we will feel, and the more easily we can entertain our brain cells with Healthy Fixes instead. You'll spend time studying yourself and listing the most potent triggers and then instituting plans to rid yourself of them.

You'll also learn how to use emergency "safe highs," whole food combinations that will hit all the sweet/salty/fatty notes you need yet won't allow you to come within 10 feet of foods you abuse. And while I want you to get moving, there's no "feeling the burn" in this stage! Extreme exercise lowers the level of acetylcholine, a neurotransmitter that helps prevent relapse and sensitivity to rebound cravings. Instead, you'll start out slow and steady, with rhythmic cardiovascular exercises that keep acetylcholine levels stable while they warm up the hypothalamus and increase the brain's release of soothing, calming serotonin, nature's antidepressant.

You'll learn dozens of other Mind, Mouth, and Muscle strategies to interrupt the False Fix cycle as soon as possible—preferably before it even starts—and immediately replace it with another reward, *right away*. You're reclaiming your reward system.

Stage 2: Beginner Recovery: Strengthening the PFC

Once you've shown you have made the Healthy Fix behavioral and lifestyle changes and have reached your Detox goal, you'll transition into Stage 2. This is where you lay the foundation for a successful lifelong recovery from food addiction. In this stage, you'll spend lots of time practicing, refining, and honing the basic skills and techniques you learned in Detox. Behavioral change takes time, and you've got endless time opportunities in this stage. You'll have the option to practice smart relapses, and you may have to circle back to Detox if life hits and you fall off the wagon. No worries. I've got your back. Stage 2 is where you practice, practice, practice. And then, one magical day, you've built enough new neural circuits in your brain that when a False Fix rears its ugly head, your new normal knee-jerk reaction is to shout "NO!" and refuse the seduction.

Think of those poor junk-food-craving rats we discussed earlier—they were *miserable* without their fatty food, but they didn't know any other way. They tried to resist the healthy food because they wanted to feel the high they got with the junk. But they were able to make it back to a place where their brains recovered and they could eat the healthy food again. And the good news is that you can successfully adapt as well.

Remember what Charles Darwin once said: "It is not the strongest of the species that survives, nor the most intelligent that survives. It is the one that is the most adaptable to change." The secret to successful survival is the ability to adapt and adjust to life's stresses without resorting to self-destruction. The human body is in a constant, dynamic state of adapting and adjusting, increasing or decreasing protein secretion, receptor sensitivity, endocrine secretion, and more. It's the repeated exposures and habits that drill in significant subconscious habitual behaviors, such as always stopping at a red light.

During Stage 2, we do everything we can to toughen up your sensitive PFC. Consider it your executive center boot camp. Every time you resist your False Fix and choose a Healthy Fix instead, you are building stamina by tapping the mesocortical dopamine system in the prefrontal cortex, an area more involved in motivation, organization, and attention. This stage is where you slug it out, day after day, long after the honeymoon phase of 4 weeks or so is over. You're learning what it's going to be like to live a life of successful recovery from food addiction.

Research on opioid addicts has found that when the addicts are done with their withdrawal and are out of rehab, they can experience a prolonged period of sadness, withdrawal, depression, and feeling physically bad—until they are given drugs that boost their serotonin. Not surprisingly, your PFC also loves and thrives on plenty of serotonin. So in our quest to strengthen the PFC in Stage

2, we'll provide you as many natural sources of serotonin as we can.

Stress can have a significant impact on PFC functioning. Studies using fMRI have shown that simply reducing stress can enhance the functioning back up to the level of other nonstressed people. That's why radical stress reduction remains a top priority,[7] especially through meditation and body movement. Meditation, and specifically Transcendental Meditation (TM), has been shown to significantly augment PFC function. And regular physical activity increases the body's production of brain-derived neurotrophic factor, or BDNF, a protein that stimulates new growth in several areas of your brain—including that precious PFC.

In Stage 2, you are working to achieve your goal weight—but it's *not* just about body weight. Instead, we're aiming for optimal body composition. By monitoring your body fat percentage, you can make sure you're not dropping lean or muscle mass. You're staying physically fit by building and preserving lean body mass while shedding overall weight.

Through it all, we'll constantly reflect upon your EpiphaME—the motivation and meaning that have become your mental anchor in a stormy sea. Discipline alone will never succeed. The greater the hunger you feel about your quest to control your food addiction, the less discipline is needed to carry out your program. The journey becomes joyful and pleasurable even when most challenging. Reward gives discipline a purpose.

Stage 3: Master Recovery: Slipping into Your Skinny Genes

The golden question remains: How can we make sure these positive changes are permanent? And how can we reverse some of the negative damage we've already done?

Thankfully, your epigenetics has been improving with every step of the Hunger Fix lifestyle, through each action taken. The proteins surrounding each gene, the histones, are constantly monitoring all actions as well as any influence from the physical environment. Based on your choices, your genes have started a domino effect—and what was once a trend in the negative direction has certainly changed course by now. When you used to eat Ho Hos, you created one kind of epigenetic change; now that you eat an apple, you create the opposite.

Your genes now *are* your environment—there is no difference because your genes and your environment are so intimately interconnected. Prior genetic expression may remain at some level, like a residual old habit lurking in the shadows ready to express itself should you enable the False Fixes to emerge once again. This is why addictions never completely disappear. Vigilance—a key outcome of good PFC function—is absolutely critical for the rest of an addict's life. Stage 3's focus is squarely on protecting your lifelong practice of Healthy Fixes to quell the deeply embedded urges.

When you first started Detox, you were fragile. *Can I make it? Will I be able to fulfill my dreams?* In Stage 3, you celebrate as a master, someone who has toughed it out and is now reaping the rewards, the authentic natural dopamine-driven rewards of a Healthy Fix lifestyle. In Stage 3, committing yourself to a new challenge is much less daunting than it once would have been. At this point, you are so immersed in the rewards of Healthy Fixes that you truly recognize that the best, most enjoyable life you can lead will be a continual process of reward refinement. You will look around, see the new landscape of your life, and decide, "What's next? How can I keep this going?" Now's when you'll set your sights on goal you might not have ever dreamed possible:

Finish a 10-K—or a triathlon!

Start your own business.

Hike the Grand Canyon.

Bicycle around Europe.

Learn how to tango.

Post your sexy new profile picture on Match.com.

Seem big? You bet. But here's your ace in the hole: In addition to affecting pleasure and motivation, dopamine is also the neurotransmitter of *achievement*. The act of successfully sticking to your plan will have become a Healthy Fix in itself. No one can expect to eliminate *all* False Fixes—indeed, perfectionism is a False Fix!—but if you're really listening to your new Healthy Fix brain, you'll *need* to "do" that Healthy Fix all over again and again and again.

How Long Will This Take?

Short answer? Entirely up to you. Your Hunger Fix program is 100 percent determined by your own pace and progress. Nora Volkow, MD, director of the National Institute on Drug Abuse, says that for recovery programs be effective, they really have to be 90 days or longer. A 30-day period does not appear to be sufficient for people with a severe addiction problem. At 90 days, you start to significantly improve the outcomes.

I have seen the most success when patients stick with Detox for at least 3 to 4 weeks (longer if they're still feeling out of control) and then remain in Stage 2 until they reach and maintain 80 percent of their body composition goal for 6 months. That PFC practice, practice, practice takes time—and even then, you'll be in Stage 3 for the rest of your life—so what's your hurry?

Are you ready to take yourself on? Now it's time to experience your EpiphaME!

CHAPTER 4

The EpiphaME: Finding Your True Hunger

GRATITUDE BESTOWS REVERENCE, ALLOWING US
TO ENCOUNTER EVERYDAY EPIPHANIES, THOSE
TRANSCENDENT MOMENTS OF AWE THAT CHANGE
FOREVER HOW WE EXPERIENCE LIFE AND THE WORLD.
—JOHN MILTON

I RUSHED INTO MY OFFICE ONE DAY, AND AS I WHIZZED past the door to the waiting room, I spotted a petite blond who looked like a fitness trainer. I wondered who had referred her and why she was there. Soon enough, Anne was getting comfortable in her chair in my office. I glanced at the chart and saw that her main complaint was stomach upset. Looking up, I smiled as Anne began reciting her amazing story.

A successful entrepreneur, Anne dropped back from full-time to part-time daily business operations once she became pregnant, while her husband assumed a larger leadership role. She thrust herself into motherhood with the same passion and vigor she had when she started her company years earlier. And like so many women, she became the ultimate caregiver to everyone but herself. Stress and the growing realization that her marriage was not working took their toll—her weight skyrocketed.

Before Anne knew it, the extra pounds had transformed into serious obesity. Her 5-foot-1-inch frame struggled under the burden of 250 pounds. Doctors harped about her medical risk as blood sugars, cholesterol, and blood pressure shot through the roof. Too busy and dissociated to want to hear any of it, Anne just kept getting an A+ as a mom and professional and an F- in tending to her own needs.

Flash forward a decade. At the age of 40, Anne found herself weeping by the bedside of her best friend, who was dying of cancer. Her friend had always taken good care of herself and had outlasted the dire prognosis by 2 years. Yet here she was, in her final days.

And then it happened: Anne thought, "There are *no* options for my beloved friend. But here I sit with my whole life in front of me. My God, what have I done to myself? I have options and I'm wasting my life carting around all of this fat that brings me down and interferes with my dreams. I damned well know what to do." As her eyes filled with tears, she vowed to turn her life around.

After the funeral, Anne didn't miss a beat. She toughed out the weeks of junk-food withdrawal, joined a gym, and began her new life. Was it easy? Hell, no. As she closely examined the persons, places, and things in her life, she realized that many of them didn't support her new lifestyle. The stomach upset that brought her to me was associated with the stress of the adaptations and adjustments she was making to create a new life for herself. It meant making critical and painful decisions about what worked and didn't work in her life.

And that included her husband.

Despite extraordinary challenges and endless emotional roller coasters, Anne realized the anchor that kept her steady in these stormy waters was that one moment when she sat with her dying friend and realized she had to change.

Two years later and 130 pounds lighter, Anne has emerged as one of my most avid Peeke Performers, a burgeoning athlete, a cyclist. When she competes, she writes her friend's name on her race bib to remind her, once again, how in the waning hours of a young woman's life another life had been born. And for that, Anne is eternally grateful for the gift of her EpiphaME.

EpiphaME is my term for a sudden, mind-blowing, sometimes life-changing insight into some essential meaning in your own reality. It's a monumental moment for any food addict.

The process of change most frequently requires some kind of wake-up call, anything from a life-threatening close call to a marital mishap to a sudden rebirth of vanity. One of my most successful patients dropped more than 120 pounds because of her first thought when she won a lifetime achievement award in her field. She realized, "I'll be damned if I'm going to allow how I look and feel about myself ruin this incredible day." That was 10 years ago. Since then, she's managed to keep her food addiction at bay—exactly the same way you will.

Kicking food addiction is hard. You need fuel for the journey. That fuel is your true hunger—the passion that drives you to pay attention to yourself, the motivation that inspires you, the goal you can see with crystal clarity; in other words, what your soul really aches for instead of the food coma. Your Healthy Hunger. And you find that hunger within your EpiphaME.

Like Anne, you need to really look at how you live and why it's been so hard for you to stop your self-destructive habits. Many people on False Fixes see the world in their own way. Your False Fixes may "work" for you because you fear the price of change. You might feel you don't deserve more. Over time, your brain adapted to what it perceives as your "normal" state.

Your False Fixes could include a bad marriage that makes you angry and depressed—so you self-destruct by eating junk, not taking care of yourself, not seeing your friends.

Your False Fixes could include a dead-end job that drains you emotionally, leaving you feeling helpless, hopeless, and defeated. So you eat to numb the pain you feel just thinking about going to work.

Your False Fix could be loneliness, so you spend night after night on the computer or watching TV and living vicariously through other people's lives, willing your food coma to anesthetize you from your pain.

Or your False Fix could be a frenetic 24/7 lifestyle where you have to schedule bathroom breaks and leave no room to care for yourself. You dashboard dine, mindlessly eating anything that's not tacked down—and, once again, the science fair projects you stick in your mouth take on a life of their own.

You keep living like this. Not even a front-end loader can get you up in the morning. Your insomnia stimulates hunger hormones, creating biological confusion and pushing you to keep reaching for food in a desperate search for satisfaction. But nothing seems to work.

So you wake up, don't exercise, skip breakfast, and end up throwing big cash away at the coffee place, on a gigundo triple-caffeinated sugary drink and monster muffin. You wear the same huge black-brown-navy hide-it clothes, day after day.

You're addicted to the flood of pleasure from these faux foods, the resulting trance. You become as addicted to the ritual of eating these foods as you are addicted to the druglike foods themselves. The drive-thru has become your dealer; the straw in the soda is your syringe.

Why do you continue to live like this? Because somehow it works for you. The effects are familiar and comfortable. Your False Fixes are the fake, comfortable, secure rewards associated with these habits.

No change in life ever happens unless the old sources of quick-hit–quick-drop dopamine are supplanted by newer, more attractive, more sustainable sources—and you can *never* make that happen without a major mind shift. Ah, but how to get one of those?

They are possible, you know. Chances are you've already experienced one in another sector of your life.

Many women find that at one distinct moment in their lives, they can easily give up smoking and drinking, eat well and get proper sleep, walk every day, and stay relaxed—no problem! When do they achieve this miraculous shift in self-care?

You guessed it: When they're pregnant. They know every choice they make while pregnant has a direct impact on their baby. And they *hunger* for a healthy baby.

Somehow parents seem to manage to do for their kids what they cannot find the strength to do for themselves. Even if you are not a parent, you must care for yourself as if you were. Your challenge is to make that same resolution for yourself, to make the connection between your day-to-day actions and choices and an ultimate reward that is deeply and personally meaningful to you—your Healthy Hunger. The pint of ice cream looks less appealing once you realize your dream job promotion depends upon your appearing fit and healthy. That box of cookies loses its magnetic pull when you're warned that you're *this close* to being diabetic and if you don't change your ways, you will have to swallow a slew of pills and eventually inject yourself with insulin.

An EpiphaME gets your attention so you can regroup, home in on your Healthy Hunger, and get started on your food addiction recovery. I have spent thousands of hours working with men and women, helping them uncover their game-changing EpiphaME. And once that occurs, magic happens.

Once you've found your EpiphaME, suddenly your mind shifts. And all the BMW—bitch, moan, whine—about the loads of work involved with losing weight comes to a grinding halt. Your mind and body dissociation—"Problem, *what* problem?"—evaporates. You're fully aware, mindful, and in the present. Your brain has fixated on the new, bigger reward.

Change occurs once you perceive that the work involved with improving your life is finally less than the work it's taking to maintain your present state of being. When you see that the reward for achieving your Healthy Hunger far exceeds the reward for staying hooked on your False Fixes—and you are willing to do the work. The EpiphaME helps to connect you to your raw, naked, and authentic self.

Anatomy of an EpiphaME

Your EpiphaME is like a "click" goes off in your brain. Suddenly you can no longer stand the thought of wearing the dreary hide-it clothes. You rustle up the nerve to join the gym and sign up for a spin class. You're filled with a fierce determination to end what is now pain and angst. Your eyes are wide open. You can see the lie.

Your dreams and aspirations become wrapped around substituting Healthy Fixes for your former False Fixes. You develop a False Fix radar. You start scanning your environment and habits, becoming acutely aware of their presence. Your dopamine system is geared up to give you pleasure with every pound of mental and physical weight removed, with every inch that disappears, with every new piece of smaller clothing you wear. Your malleable PFC is developing new neuronal circuits to support these new behaviors. Old excuses fall by the wayside. Patience, perseverance, and practice seal the deal.

One of my favorite examples of an EpiphaME came from a patient whose former doctor had uttered two simple words. Joann was 100 pounds overweight, sitting on the examination table in her paper gown, waiting for her physical exam. Her primary care doctor walked in. He looked at her and simply asked, "Still fat?"

That was it. She could taste her anger as she left that day. Her next stop was my office.

Fourteen months later, she had removed 100 pounds. She walked into her primary care physician's office for an exam, but she never undressed.

He came into the exam room and was visibly shocked. She smiled and said, "Thanks for getting me so pissed off I finally was knocked into reality. However, your crass and rude way of dealing with me has led me to come here today to terminate my relationship with you. You're fired!"

And with that, she left. She's kept the weight off for 10 years. Now, that's the best revenge!

Your EpiphaME Is Key to Long-Term Change

There is a saying, "If you love what you do, you will never work a day in your life."

If you have a real EpiphaME, you will not need external forces screaming at you to do the right thing. Instead, you'll draw from a positive, powerful place deep inside of you. Suddenly it is easier and makes complete sense to simply do the right thing and not turn life into an endless nightmare boot camp.

Reward now becomes the central factor: "What's in it for me?"

Let's say you want to drop some weight for your wedding. You'd love to show off a smaller waist in your gown on your special day.

Now, we know that having a smaller waist decreases your risks of heart disease, cancer, depression, and diabetes. But for your purposes, you don't care about that—you just want to look good! Well, consider this: A study from the University of Liverpool using fMRI scans of men found heightened activity in guys' nucleus accumbens, the forebrain area highly involved in reward processes, when they saw images of women with a low waist-to-hip ratio—aka the hour-glass figure.[1] That's right—men's brains literally get their fix just from the sight of a nice curvy body with a small waist, likely because it is an evolutionary signal for heightened fertility.

Who doesn't want to be craved like a drug by their partner? You're hooked on health, he's hooked on you. Heck—you're both high! Not a bad way to start out your married life together.

The EpiphaME is the tipping point, the moment rich with the promise of newer, more seductive, and powerful rewards. And these rewards, these Healthy Hungers, are unique to the individual:

> Zipping yourself up into sexy smaller jeans with a tucked-in white blouse
>
> Not having to shop in Lane Bryant or the Big Man department
>
> Knocking the socks off your ex-boyfriend or girlfriend at the reunion
>
> Getting off the meds
>
> Making your kid proud
>
> Getting the promotion
>
> Running that 5-K

While these Healthy Hungers take work to achieve, some EpiphaMEs occur with lightning speed—one word, a certain look, an event. Others develop over time—you read the article that inspires you, but you don't take action. You're thinking about joining a gym. You're not there yet, but you're getting closer. When you finally realize what it is you are *really* getting—and not getting—from your False Fixes, that's when the healing can begin.

Mitch wanted to drop 50 pounds. He's a superachieving psychologist who works too many hours—work is his whole life. He finds it hard to say no—except to his own workouts and healthy eating. Mitch has always suffered from anxiety, depression, and self-doubt. His mother

(continued on page 68)

Are You Ready?

Have you already had your EpiphaME, or do you still need one?

	Yes	No
1. Are you motivated to make long-term lifestyle changes that require eating healthy foods and becoming more physically active?		
2. Have you fully identified the main stresses in your life now and during the next several months?		
3. Do you truly believe that there is no magic bullet, but instead patient work on your part?		
4. Do you believe that you can change your eating habits?		
5. Do you have family, friends, or both who will support your weight-loss efforts?		
6. Are you willing to find ways to be more physically active?		
7. Are you realistic about your mental and physical transformation goal?		
8. Are you willing to record your food intake, physical activity, and mental focus, and will you make time to do so?		
9. Are you willing to look at past experiences in starting a healthier lifestyle and other areas of your life to see what has motivated you and kept you working on obstacles to success?		
10. Do you view changing your eating and physical activity habits as a positive experience?		
11. Have you resolved, or are you in the process of resolving, any eating disorders or other emotional issues that make it difficult for you to achieve a healthy weight?		
12. Do you believe that achieving your mental and physical transformation is a lifelong process that requires you to change your behavior, eating habits, and level of physical activity?		
13. Are you ready to make that commitment?		

Scoring Key

0: Precontemplation: Are you sure you're *really* reading this book? Just kidding. Not to worry—you'll get there. As of now, you're still completely happy with your False Fixes—they're your best friends. You sink into that food coma every day. Nothing is wrong. Ignorance is bliss. "I don't have a problem." As you chomp on another cookie or candy or bag of chips, you think, "I probably shouldn't be doing this," but you continue anyway. You're just becoming aware of a little nagging whisper of a voice in your head that's saying, "Are you sure you want to do that?"

1–3: Contemplation: You're reading this, but you're not sold. You're still holding back. You hate your False Fixes, but getting rid of them is such a pain in the ass. You're all BMW—bitch, moan, whine: "It would be so hard. I don't wanna." Or "I'm going to do it at some point—just not now." However, that nagging whisper is getting louder. You're reading more articles about how to change up your habits in magazines, in the newspaper, and on the Web. You're beginning to observe the habits of people who seem to have it together and aren't hooked on False Fixes. There's a battle waging in your head between the BMW voices and those encouraging you to dream and hope for freedom from your False Fixes.

4–6: Preparation: You're ready. You get it. You've found your EpiphaME. You see the end goal. You really want to change. You're already thinking about what you're going to do. Maybe you've even made a few rules for yourself, like no more refined carbs or no eating before bed. You're starting to get excited—change is coming soon.

7 or More: Action: You have a pencil in your hand and you're taking notes. You plan to get to work the second you close the cover of this book. You threw out all your False Fix foods 3 days ago. You are a walking EpiphaME. And *this* is where your Healthy Fix lifestyle program begins.

brutalized him with harsh criticism and demands for most of his life. One of his False Fixes is thinking she has control over him. One of his Healthy Fixes is his family—he has a great wife and kids. He "does" his False Fixes of cookies and sugar when he's stressed and anxious.

During our work together, he finally stepped back and found the source of the domino effect—what started what. He had given his mother power over him. His endless work schedule was his attempt to overcompensate for the feelings of self-worth he lacked based on his rough upbringing. Once his angst and anger had reached a critical level, he could make finally make changes.

Boom! He got it. "I'm not going to allow her or anyone else to control me any longer. I want to be free, and I suddenly realized only I hold the key to my freedom."

He made time for the trainer and the gym and more vacations with family. He dropped weight. His reward system transitioned into one of joy for a body and mind that felt happiness he never knew existed.

This major mind change occurs when *the pain of where you are now is far greater than the pain it will take to get out.* You crave your Healthy Hunger. The rewards have shifted to favor the Healthy Fix.

You will keep this Healthy Hunger front and center, and your entire program will nurture and strengthen it while you withdraw from your False Fixes. As you go on, your Healthy Hunger may change over time. What was a major driver today may be supplanted by another based on a new life experience. What gets you started—your EpiphaME— will always stick with you. But what keeps you going for a lifetime— your Healthy Hunger—may be something entirely different.

A retired military nurse, Judy gained 50 pounds in the 4 years since she'd left the army. Having battled depression and insomnia most of her life, Judy realized that her feelings of hopelessness and defeat were stimulating her appetite and packing on the pounds. Her EpiphaME smacked her in the head one day as she cared for her dying father in his home. As she tried to move him onto his side to change a wound dressing, she complained to her mother that even with his profound weight loss, he was quite heavy to move around. Curious, she looked at his medical records to read his weight. Reading "160," she dropped the chart. "My God, that's *my* weight, too!" But that's where the similarities stopped. He was 5 foot 10; she was 5 foot 1.

"How did I end up weighing the same as my dad? And if he feels so heavy, I do, too!" She could almost feel the mental click in her head. "I'm way out of control. I just can't believe what's happened to me."

Still stunned by this revelation, she attended one of my Peeke Week Retreats at Red Mountain Spa in St. Georges, Utah. There she started a new chapter in her life. Her "I cannot believe I weigh the same as my dad" EpiphaME soon evolved into a surprising new Healthy Hunger— "I've got to stay on track for my next triathlon." Yep, Judy resurrected her lifelong love of swimming and added biking and running. She became one of my Peeke Performers and had a new way to stay accountable, vigilant, and on track with her Healthy Fix lifestyle.

The stronger the resolve and reward, the less painful the process. If you've taken the "Are You Ready?" quiz, but you're not at the preparation or action stage, try the following exercise. Sometimes this helps my patients to see the way that they are holding themselves back.

Creating Your Own EpiphaME

"He who has a *why* can endure any *how*."

Nietzsche may have said it first, but scientists have long since proved it. One NYU study showed that having a meaningful longer-range goal made people more likely to resist immediate gratification, increased their physical endurance, boosted confidence in their ability to resist temptation, and even decreased the lure of the temptations themselves.[2] If you are out of shape and unfit, a number on a scale will just *never* be the driver for your goal. You need to drop mental weight before you can drop the physical weight. You have to zero in on the real goal, because inside that goal is a Healthy Hunger you can feel. You want it so badly you can just *taste* it.

In this exercise, I want you to go deep and identify an elemental need that stings, one that is so meaningful that you can taste the reward already. That need will help you identify a Healthy Hunger reward strong enough to bring forth your EpiphaME. And by identifying your positive and negative habits around that goal, you can see the persons, places, and things that will facilitate or impede the achievement of the goal.

COLUMN 1. IDENTIFY AN IMPORTANT HEALTHY FIX

To help you pinpoint a change you'd really like to accomplish and that has meaning to you, ask yourself the following questions: What is one habit that bothers me and is also one that is not impossible to change? Based on these answers, what am I really hungering to achieve in my life?

Let's say you really want the energy to keep up with all of your

1. My Healthy FIX	2. Things I Do to Hinder My Healthy FIX	3a. Fears and Worries
Eat a nutritious breakfast.	Get to bed late. Wake up tired and rushed. Fail to plan. Don't get to the grocery store on time. Keep the kitchen packed with junk food. Eat at my desk. Skip breakfast altogether.	I probably won't stick to it. My spouse/kids like junk food. My spouse will be angry with the new sleep schedule. I'll lose control with a False Fix. **3b. Commitments and Obligations** I am committed to a regular habit of having a healthy breakfast every morning, and I am proud of my efforts to accomplish this goal. I am committed to establishing a healthier eating routine for my family and myself through consistent education and the substitution of tasty Healthy Fixes for the junk and False Fixes currently in my home.

activities and derive more joy from living life to the fullest. You identify that you eat junk food all day and this contributes to your lack of energy and focus. So your Healthy Fix is to eat a nutritious breakfast to fuel you properly at the start of each day. (Be sure to create a simple, doable action that you can stick to, and enter this in column 1.)

COLUMN 2. TAKE RESPONSIBILITY FOR YOUR ROLE

It's time to tell the truth about your typical habits. Look at the Healthy Fix you have chosen. Now think of all of the habits you currently practice that interfere with incorporating your Healthy Fix in your life. Make a list and don't censor. Just let your thoughts rip and write everything that comes to mind. Enter that list into column 2.

COLUMN 3A. FILL IN YOUR FEARS

People fear failure. They also fear what will happen if they *do* change. How will your life change if you're successful? Will others support your new lifestyle, or might they feel alienated by your actions or not want to participate? Close your eyes and imagine you have succeeded. Let's say you are able to have a nutritious breakfast every morning. You might worry that you won't stick to it, or that your family may resent the fact that you want to swap out junk food for healthier options. No matter what your fears are, articulating them is a valid and important step in realizing what it will take to create a Healthy Fix.

Write those fears into the Fear and Worries box.

COLUMN 3B. DETERMINE THE COMMITMENTS AND OBLIGATIONS THAT COMPETE WITH YOUR HEALTHY FIX

Instead of considering your fears and worries as impediments to success, you're now going to do something different. Turn each fear inside out and transform it into a commitment to make certain that this fear never happens. You're being proactive and protecting your ability to achieve your Healthy Fix habit by giving yourself a heads-up for potential problems. In column 3b, transform your fears into a commitment that will allow you to begin and practice your Healthy Fix habit.

Again, using the example above, the fear and concern that "I probably won't stick to it" becomes the statement: "I am committed to a regular habit of having a healthy breakfast every morning, and I am proud of my efforts to accomplish this goal." Similarly, "My spouse/kids like junk food in the house and won't let me clean things up and get rid of the stuff" now becomes "I am committed to establishing a healthier eating routine for my family and myself, through consistent education and the substitution of tasty Healthy Fixes for the junk and False Fixes currently in my home."

Now pause for a moment and look at what you've written in these three columns. To the left, you see a Healthy Fix you hunger for. In the middle, you see your own current behaviors—and it's clear how they will hinder achieving your Healthy Fix goal. And to the right, you come face-to-face with your fears and worries about how your life will change if you start to practice and live your Healthy Fix habit. Then you see how to invert each fear into a proactive commitment freeing you to achieve your Healthy Fix goal.

Many patients find this exercise uncovers their EpiphaME as well as refines it. It's an important first step to overcoming your resistance to change and helping you move forward to your true reward, your Healthy Hunger. You can see, in black and white, "What's in it for me?"

Feeling Your Healthy Hunger

Once you think you have your EpiphaME, let's see if your Healthy Hunger is strong enough to hold up under fire during your typical day. Do this simple exercise. Let's say that your EpiphaME reads like this: "I'm totally freaked out. Just found out I'm prediabetic. I never

ever want to have to inject myself with a needle so I will absolutely change my diet and start exercising." Your Healthy Hunger becomes "I want to get so healthy I never have to see a syringe!"

Now write down your Healthy Hunger and keep it front and center throughout your busy day. Keep a reminder everywhere you can—next to the toothbrush, on your fridge, as a screensaver on your computer.

Next, go through your usual day and be very observant about what happens to your Healthy Hunger focus when you're tired, beat up, homicidal, and completely overwhelmed right around 3:00 or 4:00 p.m., when you feel drawn to the reward of that False Fix to numb you. Is your Healthy Hunger strong enough to snap you out of your food trance and get you past the danger zone? How about when you get home at night, during dinner, or when you're getting the after-dinner stirrings for a False Fix or two. Is your Healthy Hunger hanging in there?

If it's not, no worries. Simply go back to the "Creating Your Own EpiphaME" exercise and keep working it, rewriting the Healthy Fixes and delving into your real true needs, and then experiment to see if that's the anchor to keep you focused throughout the day.

Now that you have locked in your reward, you're ready to commit. Let's gather some more information that will help you launch into Stage 1: Detox on the right foot.

Create your Hunger Fix video journal. To lock in the feeling of this EpiphaME, I want you to journal. But not journal in the way that you used to—I want you to sit in front of your computer, your smartphone, or your digital camera and record your own personal Hunger Fix video journal.

In each step of the Hunger Fix program, you're going to use this video journal to lock in and lock down your rewards. In each installment, you will speak to your future self, to remind that person what False Fixes have done to your life and why you want to change them. Get emotional if you want. Scream, rant, and rave. Or sit quietly and thoughtfully as you tell your truth. You'll continue with the Hunger

Fix video journal throughout the program as a progress tracker. More so than a snapshot, a video can be a powerful, visceral reminder of where you started and how far you've come.

For this first installment, I'd like you to talk about what has brought you to this moment. Recall any of the most challenging times you fully experienced your own weight, and describe the experiences in as graphic detail as you possibly can: "Why am I doing this? What am I walking away from? What am I walking toward?" If you have it, state your EpiphaME and Healthy Hunger loud and clear. Stop taping, hit rewind, and listen to yourself. This first video journal entry will be a priceless anchor to remind you why this is a lifesaving journey.

Gather your False Fix health history. The more you can look at where you've been, the clearer a path you can create for where you're going. Collect your personal health information in one place, so you can really face it.

Epigenetic Profile

1. Age, height, and current weight.

2. Occupation.

3. Your marital status (married, divorced, living with someone, widowed, single, separated).

4. If applicable, the age, height, current weight, and occupation of your "significant other."

5. If you have children, list the age and gender of each child and note if the child has any addictive behaviors and/or history of being under- or overweight.

6. List any current prescription medications you are taking, for what purpose, and how long you have been taking them.

7. List any over-the-counter medications and/or dietary supplements (vitamins, minerals, herbs, etc.) you are currently taking, for what purpose, and how long you have been taking them.

8. List any known allergies to food or medications.

9. List any past and/or current medical problems, i.e., heart disease, diabetes, high blood pressure, depression.

10. List any hospitalizations, with dates.

11. Family addiction history: List any family members with a history of addictions. Note what kind(s) of addiction(s):
    a. Overweight or obesity
    b. Eating disorders
    c. Heart disease
    d. Diabetes
    e. Cancer
    f. Other:

12. Personal addiction history: Do you have a history of addictions? Note what kind(s) of addiction(s):
    a. Overweight or obesity
    b. Eating disorders
    c. Heart disease
    d. Diabetes
    e. Cancer
    f. Other:

13. Environmental addiction history:
    a. Do you live with anyone with any form of addiction? If so, please note what kind(s) of addiction(s).
    b. Do you live or work in an environment with individuals who have a history of addiction(s)?

14. Starting with childhood, summarize your weight history, including your weight/size during childhood, high school, college, graduate school, and for each 5 years thereafter.

15. Chart your weight over time, including weight, year, and any milestone/event (include onset or termination of any addiction) that influenced the weight at that time (see page 76):

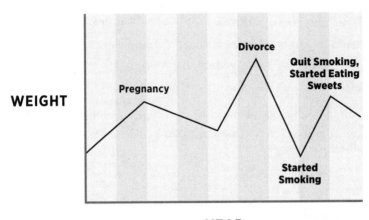

WEIGHT

Pregnancy

Divorce

Quit Smoking,
Started Eating
Sweets

Started
Smoking

YEAR

16. List any methods you have used in the past for weight management.

17. Describe your typical weekday schedule, beginning with the time you awaken, your daytime and nighttime activities, eating, exercise, and the time you go to bed. When describing your eating patterns, please provide the typical foods eaten at the time you have a meal or snack.

18. List any foods that make you feel you lose control and overeat/ binge. (Note: You'll take another quiz about this in a minute.)

19. Over the course of a week, how often do you make time to exercise?

20. Sleep history:

    a. On average, how many hours do you sleep?

    b. Do you have trouble getting to sleep or staying asleep?

Take the Yale Food Addiction Scale Survey. If you're curious to see if you truly qualify as a food addict, take the only scientifically validated tool to measure food addiction, created by Ashley Gearhardt of Yale (see Appendix A on page 303). If you meet the criteria described, then you do have a food addiction. The test was based on the criteria for substance abuse as stated in the Diagnostic and Statistical Manual of Mental Disorders IV-R (DSM-IVR), and it measures your addiction on several scales.

Take a False Fix food inventory. Sit down with two pieces of paper. Fold the sheets in half lengthwise.

1. Down the left-hand side of one sheet, write the foods you eat all the time, as well as the quantities. Most people stick to a limited rotation of foods—maybe 10 dinners that they rotate over and over. Healthy foods, unhealthy foods—whatever you eat on a regular basis, write down what and how much. Circle the foods that you wish you could eat less of.

2. Then, on the left side of the *second* piece of paper, write down all the foods you ate on the worst days of eating you've ever had. Just try your best to recall. Maybe it was stuffed French toast for breakfast, a supersize fast-food meal for lunch, and half a pizza on your own for dinner. Maybe it was a five-scoop sundae—after you'd already scarfed down a burger, fries, and a soda. A session with spinach and artichoke dip? Church basement supper of casseroles galore? The idea here is not to think about what you might ordinarily eat but to recall what you have eaten in one big day. Dig deep. Whatever it was, just lay it all out there.

3. Now, with the first list in hand, take out a calorie counter or go to a Web site like www.calorieking.com. Write down how many grams of fat and carbs and how many calories are in every serving. Then multiply by the number of servings you would typically have. For example, take out a ½-cup measuring cup; look at it and think about your last plate of pasta. A typical box of pasta has eight servings in it. How many servings did you eat last time? Write down the calorie total for each dish.

4. Do the same calorie count for your "worst day ever" list.

5. Stare at those numbers. Really see them. Try to absorb the reality of the caloric load you've been putting in your body. Welcome to sticker shock.

If you're reading this and thinking to yourself, "Oh, I don't have to do this—I know what I've been eating," please, I beg of you, don't skip this step. This exercise is a mindblower for all my patients. You *must* relive the binges and bouts of overeating to thoroughly understand how much power your False Fixes have had over you.

I think of this like a DUI blood alcohol content number—it's an objective gauge of how out of control you were with your False Fixes. One of my patients said, "I started to understand exactly what each of those False Fixes 'cost me'—knowing that information really helped me make better, clearer choices."

Part of the EpiphaME is to confront precisely what you were doing. When we decide to change and concentrate *only* on the positive future, thinking about how many calories are in string beans, we miss the lesson of where we've been. You need to truly understand that you were consuming 2,000 calories at a pop during a dinner you wouldn't even consider a "binge." This False Fix EpiphaME is about facing the demons and understanding thoroughly what you're choosing to avoid for the rest of your life.

Identify your motivation mantra. You need a way to maintain your connection with your anchoring Healthy Hunger. Create a simple, easy-to-remember phrase (or even a number) that will be your constant companion. You could choose words that resonate from the Healthy Hunger exercise. Or if you're still working on discovering your Healthy Hunger, sit very still and recall the activity or experience that has given you the most joy in your life. Then think of three words to describe how you were feeling. If it's playing with your children, maybe your three words are "fun, healthy, energetic." If it's being on a trip with your significant other, maybe it's "love, bonding, adventurous." Or if it was the day your child was born, perhaps your words would be "grateful, healthy, joyous." Call on your new mantra and use it whenever cravings pop up. Counter the cravings even further with "That doesn't work for me" or "Just say no."

Clear out your cupboards. The greatest dopamine burst does not come when we eat—it comes *before* we eat. This "anticipatory reward" is the driving force of addiction—the drive to eat is the strongest part of the cycle. National Institute on Drug Abuse research and brain scans show the limbic system lights up in food addictive people when viewing foods they abuse. Keeping your trigger foods out of sight may also help keep them out of mind. Research from University of Illinois showed that when people kept chocolate inside a drawer instead of in a closed container on top of their desks, they cut their chocolate snacking by one-third without even knowing it.[3]

(I'll get more specific about purging False Fixes in Stage 1: Detox, but for now, this is a preliminary cleansing.)

1. **Toss out all False Fixes.** Throw these away, give them to a neighbor, bring them to the food pantry or church—just get them away from you, physically. They are toxic to you.

2. **Scan for sugars.** Look at the ingredient labels on all bottles, cans, and boxes. If you find high fructose corn syrup, then that container should be *gone*. Then search for anything with sugar, rice syrup, corn syrup, or an *-ose* (fructose, sucrose) as one of the first three ingredients. *Gone.*

3. **Count your ingredients.** If there are more than three ingredients that you cannot pronounce, or more than 10 ingredients total on the ingredient list, throw those foods away.

4. **Minimize your cans.** Consider replacing any canned food with frozen vegetables or dried beans. Research has linked higher concentrations of bisphenol-A (BPA) in the urine of people who eat canned foods regularly, and there was also an increased risk of cardiovascular disease and diabetes. A Harvard Study found that eating 12 ounces of soup from cans for 5 days in a row can increase the amount of BPA in your blood by 1,000 percent.[4] BPA may even affect the way nerve cells respond to dopamine and even increase the likelihood of addiction.[5] This stuff is nasty, folks—be careful.

All right, my friends. I think you are ready. It's time to detox!

CHAPTER 5

Stage 1:
False Fix Detox

THIS IS AN ADDICTION. I NEED TO STAY FOCUSED.
I NEED TO SLOW DOWN, AND THINK ABOUT WHAT I'M
GOING TO DO BEFORE I DO IT. THERE IS NO GOING BACK
TO THAT TOXIC PLACE. I'VE LEARNED A NEW WAY,
AND I KNOW THE NEW WAY WORKS FOR ME.
—DEBBY, 44, LOST 65 POUNDS IN 1 YEAR

Length of Time: 3 to 4 weeks (or more)
Detox Reward: Reduced body size; fit comfortably into Detox stage Clothes-O-Meter; elimination of False Fixes; mental calm and relaxation

WELCOME TO FALSE FIX DETOX. ARMED WITH your EpiphaME and a Healthy Hunger to achieve your dream of living the life you deserve, you're ready to start the process of mental and physical transformation.

During Detox, your brain and body need time to adapt and adjust to the new sources of dopamine and reward that come as you substitute your Healthy Fixes for False Fixes. The more you adhere to the Detox blueprint, the smoother your transition will go. This is especially true for women and men with cross-addictions, whose motivation-learning-memory reward circuits have been double and triple hijacked, and whose prefrontal cortex (PFC) has been beaten into submission. Yes, you will have to be more vigilant than someone who has one addiction (in this case, food). But I have walked many a cross-addicted individual through Detox, and with dogged determination and a passion for achieving a life worth living, they make it through to the other side.

For all of you, keep in mind that those new sources of dopamine for your brain will result in amazing rewards: strengthening your ability to focus, plan, rein in impulses, dampen any irritability and impatience, and calm you enough to make the right choices. By engaging your mind, eating Healthy Fixes, and reconnecting with your body through movement, you'll reap the priceless reward of finally feeling a sense of power over this food addiction torment.

Based on findings from the National Institute of Drug Abuse, most people will require *at least* 3 or 4 weeks to live and practice Healthy Fix habits before those habits begin to become somewhat automatic. Once you feel more energy, your sleep has improved, you are calmer, and your Clothes-O-Meter (see page 82) is looser, you'll graduate to Stage 2. On day 1 of Detox, you choose a way to document your body changes—whether it's your weight, your body composition, your measurements, or ideally, all three. (See Appendix E for more instructions.) Some people establish this baseline up front; others prefer to wait until Stage 2 to get down to the nitty-gritty of measuring results.

I want to make an important point here: We've all felt nauseated by ridiculous weight-loss claims and the myth of instant, nearly overnight weight-loss success. In the same vein, some experts claim you can "cure" your food addiction in 28 days (!) and go on to eat "just like everyone else." These, like False Fixes, are lies. As with any addiction, you must detox from the addictive substance, and thereafter you live a life of *recovery*. Beware the dangerously simplistic hype and lies about food addiction—and *don't believe them.*

Instead, believe in your own power and the power of the Hunger

Fix. I'm going to get you through your Detox and on to recovery, so you can finally live the life you deserve.

Know Your Clothes-O-Meter. Food addicts usually have spent much of their lives dissociated from their bodies. That mind-body disconnect results in a whole spectrum of self-destructive, self-denigrating attitudes and behaviors. Many of you have been so ruled by the scale that you no longer even look at your own body. In the Detox phase, reward yourself with a royal reconnection to your physical self. It's like taking a "me 101" course. But remember: "Fat talk" or negative self-speak is verboten. Detox is a terrific opportunity to learn to be gentle and kind to yourself. Banish the bashing—it's just part of the False Fix lies.

To create your Clothes-O-Meter, grab a formfitting piece of clothing—jeans, slacks, skirt, jacket, or belt—that you like but cannot comfortably wear or may not be able to put on at all. No stretchy pants, muumuus, or elastic for your Clothes-O-Meter. (When I first met one of my all-star successes, she said, "Dr. Peeke, my actual size is '*elastic.*'" She was so dissociated she lived in clothes that allowed her to float around and gain 30 pounds.) Frankly, you are more likely to be mindful and increase your sense of body awareness if you wear formfitting clothes as much as possible.

Ideally, choose clothes that require a drop of between 5 to 10 pounds to really fit well. Once you've selected your official starting Clothes-O-Meter garment, put it on (or hold it up, if it truly doesn't fit). Look in the mirror and memorize the visual—or even use your video journal to document the fit.

Put on your Clothes-O-Meter once a week and no more. Let it hang on your closet door for inspiration. Your reward is to fit into that piece of clothing by the end of your Detox. Then you'll be on your way to Stage 2.

Make a Memory. Record your day 1 of Detox in your video journal. Sit down and say out loud what your numbers are. Or just proclaim your Clothes-O-Meter goal, if that's what you're most comfortable with. Here's one example: "Hi, it's me, Sandi. Okay, this is day 1 of Detox. I'm 5 foot 6 inches and I weigh 213 pounds and my body fat is 41 percent. My tummy size is 43 inches and my hips are 46 inches. For my Clothes-O-Meter, I chose this pair of jeans that I am not ready to wear in public since they're way too tight, but I really like them. I'm hoping that in 4 weeks or so, I'll be able to zip them up!"

Then, feel free to riff away. Declare what your Healthy Hunger is: "I'm so sick and tired of living on the sidelines of my life. I want to wear a formfitting white dress at my wedding. I want to learn how to run. I *hunger* for all of this. And I'm ready to do battle with my addiction."

Cry, scream, rant, rave, calmly and lovingly talk to the camera— do whatever it takes to Detox some of these feelings right out there. The only rule is that you cannot use negative self-speak. If one of those bad boys slips out of your mouth, you must immediately say three wonderful things about yourself. Right away! You're training your brain to support you. The inner addict talk must be halted. This is your life. Live with pride. You own this journey.

Other options for day 1:

Collect some photos: Have someone take a full-body picture of you, or just reverse the camera on your smartphone and take a self-portrait. Take as many snapshots as you want, and store them in a special folder marked "Motivation." Or create a virtual scrapbook with a program such as Evernote or iDiary where you can keep the video, photos, and any text for constant reflection and progress charting. (Also, please send me your story at www.drpeeke.com. We'll post your videos, photos, and stories to inspire others on the Hunger Fix journey.)

Write it out: If you enjoy journaling, take time to write down your thoughts and feelings. Or maybe you just want to jot down a few notes per day in a weekly calendar; that's okay, too. Everyone is different, and I want to honor everyone's unique needs and approaches.

The critical point is that you document this journey. Keep shooting your videos, taking pictures, and writing throughout Detox and in Stages 2 and 3. Why? In tough times, you'll refer to your day 1 journal entry and be reminded of how far you have come. When you feel frustrated or down, you can see how much progress you've made. Way to go! Recording and documenting your journey is a priceless gift to yourself.

Neutralizing Deprivation

Normally, when people try to make a lifestyle change, they focus on what they're *not* going to do:

I'm going to stop smoking.

I'm going to stop watching TV.

I'm going to stop eating junk food.

But think of this approach through the lens of your reward system. As soon as you tell yourself, "I'm going to stop X," your brain registers that as deprivation—the absence of reward—and begins to feel stress. That stress response both mirrors and intensifies the neurochemical process of withdrawal. This vicious cycle puts you right back at the freezer door, ice-cream scoop in hand.

Instead, start at the very beginning and reframe the entire process as one gigantic ongoing parade of reward. Start this cycle with *monster* rewards in mind. Healthy, sustainable, *authentic* rewards not only help rebuild your lost dopamine receptors, but also increase the size of and strengthen your command center—the prefrontal cortex—so you'll have more brainpower to steer clear of your False Fixes and make the right choices. Don't wait until you reach your end goal to reward yourself—instead, think of every single moment of your life as an opportunity to build in another reward.

The False Fix Detox Blueprint— The Three M's

In each stage of the Hunger Fix program, you will follow a mini-plan for each of what I call the Three M's—Mind, Mouth, and Muscle. Readers of my previous books will recognize this integrative and holistic triad of behavioral domains for change. In reality, most of the Hunger Fix techniques impact all three of these domains at once. The Mind tools reinforce positive changes in Mouth and Muscle; smart Mouth choices build strong Muscle and support a healthy Mind; and so on.

MIND

MOUTH

MUSCLE

I find it helpful, at least in the beginning, to split up the Three M's so people will truly internalize that the Hunger Fix is an all-hands-on-deck task—you are going to need every piece of yourself to succeed. You'll never kick your False Fixes just by counting carbs or doing a set of leg lifts. Those are Band-Aids for bullet wounds. You have to come at your addiction with everything you have.

Stage 1: Mind focuses on destressing and anchoring your Healthy Hunger, committing to the process, and treating yourself with kid gloves so you'll have the strength to resist those foods you abuse. Stage 1: Mouth incorporates the Hunger Fix Eating Plan (see Chapters 8 and 9), which provides clear structure to support you through those first tentative weeks. I give you 28 days of breakfast, lunch, dinner, and snack options, all full of "safe highs," to help you ride out cravings by regrouping instead of relapsing. And even if you do slip, I've got your back: I teach you how to get right back on track. You'll reconnect with the pleasures of real whole foods, prepared by hand—and you'll protect your reawakening PFC by staying far away from your False Fix "foods." The Stage 1: Muscle program creates sustainable opportunities for more dopamine rushes—rhythmic, soothing ways to move your body to reawaken the pleasure of being in your own skin. (Ooh, I like the sound of that!) Remember, the goal is to teach your mind and body to create and maintain natural highs to keep the False Fixes at bay. Let's see how the Stage 1 Three M's fit together.

Stage 1: Mind

When trying to kick any False Fix, stress reduction is extremely important. And to achieve this goal, keep recalling my golden rule for survival: *When life's stresses hit, you must learn to adapt and adjust without resorting to self-destructive habits—your False Fixes.* In studies of primates without addictive genes, simply subjecting the primates to stressful social situations can reduce the number of D2 receptors in their brains and make them more susceptible to addiction. The good news is that when their stress was reduced, their D2 receptors would rebound. Researchers believe this rebound effect likely applies to humans, too.[1, 2]

Of course, a chronic high level of stress takes its toll on your body in many ways and is the driver for a number of diseases, including addiction. Corticotropin-releasing factor (CRF), a protein that triggers the release of stress hormones from your adrenal glands, seems to power the whole craving process: First, it shortens the amount of time it takes you to become addicted; then it increases the intensity of your addiction itself.[3] In a cruel catch-22, withdrawal from your False Fixes *increases* CRF-induced anxious symptoms of stress in your body—and then any excess anxiety or stress in your life will only further heighten your body's sense of withdrawal. So stress causes withdrawal, and withdrawal causes stress. The net result is a dopamine system caught in the middle, screaming out for satisfaction.[4] If you can either avoid or minimize sources of stress while you simultaneously pile on the stress-relieving Healthy Fixes, you can short-circuit both sides of this particular vicious cycle.

While we're in the Detox stage, watch out for the "three I's"—impatience, irritability, and impulsivity. As someone with a food addiction, you're used to getting your False Fix and its faux reward *right now*! Fortunately, you can learn to calm your impatience by breathing through these moments and drawing upon your new PFC-driven brainpower to stay centered and focused.

The second of the three I's, irritability, is partly based in the biology of withdrawal. You've become acclimated to specific False Fix feel-good behaviors, and suddenly they're not there. You're in a state of transition as your mind and body are adapting and adjusting to a new way of thinking, eating, and moving. I'll show you some tools and techniques to soothe your jitters and keep you on track.

Impulsive behavior, the third I, runs amuck when the PFC is weakened by chronic addiction. Some of the best interventions are those that disrupt the impulsivity that is a hallmark of addicts of all stripes. A recent article in the journal *Appetite* zeroed in on three facets of impulsivity most likely to trip up people with food addictions: lack of planning, negative mental scripts, and flash-point reactivity. We'll talk more about PFC-based planning in Stage 2. For now, in Stage 1, we'll focus on reprogramming our automatic negative reactions and mental scripts so *we* are in control, instead of our False Fixes.

First, let's start with the easy stuff: To load up on reward, you must chill.

Quash your addiction with quiet. Using your mind as command central for focus, vigilance, and stress management, you'll rein in and control your responses to life's challenges. At the same time, you'll stay calmer and better able to make productive, progressive decisions, plans and strategies. You'll feel more centered and organized.

The very first step of Detox is to find quiet time every day. Quiet time is a lifesaving, critical mental recess, a time to take a breath, rest, rejuvenate, and regroup to select the right responses to life's challenges.

Most of us have absolutely no clue how to calm our minds for an optimal quiet time. As a quadruple type A+ personality, with a mind that seemed to be missing an "off" switch, at one point, I didn't have a clue either. I thought I was chilling out on my daily runs or while hiking. Yes, it's true that exercise certainly helps us relax. But I was missing a critical element—the ability to just "be" and allow my PFC command center to operate optimally. That's when I discovered meditation.

Years ago, a wonderful friend and mentor, Dr. Herbert Benson, the founder of Harvard's Mind/Body Medical Institute, attempted to teach me his well-known relaxation response. I remember sitting in that room, closing my eyes, and lasting about 11 seconds. I was one of his most famous failures; I just didn't get it.

Over the years, I have enjoyed blissful, introspective, mindful moments, but they tended to occur in fits and spurts with no regularity. I felt like I was on a mental roller coaster, sometimes calm and centered, and other times frenzied enough to wonder if I was even born with a PFC!

Then, in the fall of 2010, my dear friend and colleague, Dr. Norm Rosenthal, sent me a review copy of his latest book, *Transcendence*. Norm is the renowned physician scientist who discovered seasonal affective disorder (SAD) and with whom I collaborated at the NIH. I read his book cover to cover and was pleasantly surprised by the groundbreaking new science associated with meditation, specifically Transcendental Meditation (TM), for which there now exists a large scientific literature. Intrigued, I decided to study this deceptively simple mental technique.

Since learning TM, I've repeatedly thought of that Zen saying, "When the student is ready, the teacher appears." Once I began my practice in earnest, I was rewarded with a remarkable experience of peace and calm, along with increased creativity, focus, and overall vigilance. And I'm in good company. My friend Dr. Mehmet Oz, Ellen DeGeneres, Paul McCartney, and Grammy Award–winning musician Moby are all TMers. Three-time Academy Award nominee and TM practitioner filmmaker David Lynch has established a foundation that has brought TM to everyone from inner city kids to traumatized soldiers (www.davidlynchfoundation.org).

You know that something's bound to get really big when Oprah embraces it as well. A recent student of TM, Oprah wrote in her *O* magazine that TM is a "powerfully energizing yet calming experience . . . I walked away feeling fuller than when I'd come in. . . . Only from that space can you create your best work and your best life."

Oprah arranged for all those interested on her staff to be taught TM, and she herself meditates once or twice a day, 20 minutes in the morning and evening. She's seen tremendous leaps in creativity and productivity among her staff, as well as other benefits, including better relationships with colleagues and loved ones, fewer headaches, and more sleep.

While TM has tremendous scientific backing, whatever form of meditation you choose will have a positive impact—as long as it involves scheduling in that quiet time and is *practiced on a consistent basis.* Think of it this way: If you want to learn how to run, you cannot do it by running once a week, then skipping a week, then running 3 days in a row, and then blowing it off for a month. You need to build strength and endurance to perform. The same holds true for your mind.

Meditation, like TM, gifts you with a "restful alertness," reducing the impulsivity that prompts you to grab for a False Fix to numb the pain of a life stress. Meditation also improves and strengthens the communication between the PFC and other parts of the brain. (We'll learn more about this in Stage 2: Beginner Recovery.) The grand result is that through regular meditative practice, you will find that your overall response to the world is calmer and more balanced.

As you progress through Detox, you may be inconsistent with your meditative practice, especially during stressful times. That's okay and expected. Kicking a False Fix is no easy job.

Meditation has always been a central focus of successful addiction recovery—it's highlighted in the 11th step of all the 12-step "Anonymous" programs (Alcoholics Anonymous, Overeaters Anonymous, and so on). The key is to jump right back on it as soon as you can.

You'll become more regular with consistent practice. We'll talk more about meditation throughout *The Hunger Fix*.

Breathe your way still. Are you like me and finding it hard to sit still for even a minute? Most people have difficulty cutting the inner mental chatter of endless worry and preworries. Here's the secret. Let your breath lead you to your center of calm. Try this easy exercise drawn from basic yoga. It's called the Pranayama, an alternate nostril breathing exercise. (*Prana* means "life force/energy," and *yama* means "discipline/control.")

First, find a place devoid of noise and sit comfortably. Then follow these steps:

1. Use your right thumb to close off your right nostril.
2. Inhale slowly through your left nostril.
3. Pause for a second.
4. Now close your left nostril with your ring finger and release your thumb off the right nostril.
5. Exhale through your right nostril.
6. Now, inhale through your right nostril.
7. Pause.
8. Use your thumb to close off your right nostril.
9. Exhale through your left nostril.

This is one round. Start slowly with 1 or 2 rounds and gradually increase if you haven't yet reached enough calm to begin your meditation. I generally need 3 or 4 rounds to reset and prepare for my twice-daily meditation practice.

> WHEN THE BREATH WANDERS, THE MIND IS UNSTEADY,
> BUT WHEN THE BREATH IS STILL, SO IS THE MIND STILL.
>
> **—HATHA YOGA PRADIPIKA**

Reach for radical relaxation. Once you've carved out some quiet time, find a stress-free haven where you can enjoy this gift of stillness.

Look for rooms, hallways, stairwells, parks, trains, or planes where no one can get to you. Turn on that PFC of yours and plot your times of relaxation throughout your day. Lock the bathroom door and take a long hot bath. Curl up and catch up on your reading.

Or you can decide to go overboard—in a good way. Scope out good deals for retreats (spa, yoga, hiking, meditation) and take a weekend or even a week off to reset and rebalance. I'm serious! By disrupting your usual habits and responses, you'll help jar your False Fix habits out of their neural grooves. Even a simple getaway to a local hotel with an indoor pool and a sauna can provide the positive disruption that kick-starts your recovery.

I know that getaways are not accessible for everyone, especially in these tough economic times. No worries! How about scheduling a massage, manicure/pedicure, or attending a restorative yoga or community center Zumba class once a week for the next 3 or 4 weeks. (Massage decreases the stress hormone cortisol by 30 percent and simultaneously raises dopamine by 30 percent—helping control both sides of the vicious False Fix cycle![5]) You have to change your routine to change your brain's knee-jerk habits. This is a critical part of addiction recovery. After putting the kids to bed, instead of doing the predictable march to the TV couch (by way of the kitchen), run to the bathroom and brush your teeth. Then draw a hot bath or take a long shower, and take a book to bed. Detox is about radical relaxation—you're resetting your body's response to stress.

Start on a Saturday. Timing is everything. The goal is to find a time in your life when you have a window of lower stress opportunity to launch your Detox. Lots of people wait until Monday to start a weight-loss program. Big mistake. Not only is Monday the most stressful day of the week, it also tends to be one of the busiest. As much as is possible, try to start Detox at a time when you don't have an abundance of competing demands. Multiple studies have shown that exerting high levels of self-control in one area of your life can make it difficult to sustain that self-control in other areas.[6] If you're in school, wait until after finals; if you're an accountant in the midst of tax season, perhaps April 16 is a better start date. Don't put off Detox for months, but be conscious about timing so you can set yourself up for success. Two days before you give a speech at the national sales conference is not the time to start kicking your False Fixes.

Create a Healthy Fix living and working environment. To ensure a successful Detox and recovery long term, you must change the way you live. Look around you. Perhaps even subconsciously, elements of your current environment are enabling and supporting your False Fixes.

People who are ensnared by their False Fix lifestyle often live and work in a state of disorganization or even cluttered chaos. As I always say, "You can't take a walk if you can't find your shoes." Rather than adopt the extremist, perfectionistic, all-or-nothing approach ("I will organize the entire house . . . today!")—as most addicts tend to do— focus on just one project a day: one shelf, one drawer, one basket. Also, change up your living space—move some furniture around! Rearrange photos, relocate plants. *Throw things away.* All of these activities delight your brain with novelty while they also break automatic responses and help your brain realize there *are* alternatives to negative patterns. An open and clean kitchen becomes a safe haven instead of crack den. Flowers by the bedside and an organized closet decrease your stress levels (and thereby control your stress-related overeating) as well as elevate your mood, keeping you focused and positive.

Please don't look at organizing as completing another boring to-do task. Instead, look at it as a stress-relieving process—you're cleaning out your head and your clutter drawer at the same time. Many addicts find the sight of one clean, organized area can be a foothold of control that will spread into other areas of life. (Check out FlyLady.net for great ideas.)

Let your False Fix go to the dogs. When we pet dogs, our blood pressure and heart rate drop, a signal that our sympathetic nervous system is taking a chill—a mini-spa break.[7] Petting a dog also decreases the stress hormone cortisol and increases plasma concentrations of dopamine, beta-endorphins, serotonin, and beta-phenylethylamine (PEA). A pleasure neurotransmitter, PEA can be raised by illicit drugs but is found in lower levels in kids with ADHD.[8] (Not surprisingly, ADHD is a major risk factor for addiction—there's that impulsivity again!)

The soft, warm touch of a pup (or a kitty) is a sensory delight, and cuddling a pet is one of the most rewarding, least demanding things we can do. A recent review article in the *Journal of Personality and Social Psychology* revealed that pet owners have better self-esteem and are less lonely, more extraverted, less fearful and neurotic, and better at handling rejection than nonpet owners.[9] The CDC also found that dog owners are 34 percent more likely to exercise for the recommended minimum of 150 minutes or more every week—a double-duty Healthy Fix![10]

Okay, so you already own three cats, two birds, or a Gila monster. Of course, many of these benefits hold true for *all* pets. The point is a wonderful pet will give you limitless, unconditional love as you journey through your Detox. And if you do choose to bring a little furry one home, be sure to do your research and think it through carefully—new puppies can create a lot of additional stress. Consider adopting an older dog: You'll be rescuing a needy animal, and you'll save yourself some of the hassle of training a young pup.

Banish False Fixes by getting out. Ecopsychologists have found that simply taking a walk outside makes stress hormone levels plummet. After time outside, both kids and adults feel more relaxed and better able to cope with their stresses. If stress levels are lower, addictive tendencies have nowhere to go. Get outside for a change of scenery that will cleanse you mentally and physically. Seek some sun—and not just in the summertime. A study published in the *Journal of Environmental Psychology* found that visiting the beach on a temperate or slightly cooler day can make the visit feel 30 percent more restorative than days that were just 3 degrees warmer.[11] Spring and fall at the beach will pack a bigger Healthy Fix punch—with cheaper hotel rates!

Get high on music. A study by McGill University found that listening to music that moves you—or even just thinking about hearing it—releases dopamine. Using PET and fMRI scans, researchers found that when people anticipate a part of the music they really enjoy, dopamine is released in the caudate in the basal ganglia, a region of the brain involved with learning and memory. But a giant surge also came at those peak moments in the song—your "favorite part!"—when a big dopamine burst is released in the nucleus accumbens, reinforcing that reward.[12] This double bang for your dopamine buck is likely what makes music such a universal part of every world culture. (Dancing with the music gives you a triple natural high!) Start making some new playlists for your commute to work or to listen to over the weekend.

OMG u r doin gr8! Throughout Detox and recovery, it's essential that you get all of the support you can (check out www.drpeeke.com). High-tech coaching—aka texting and e-mailing—definitely counts! One British study found that smokers trying to quit were twice as likely to be cigarette free after 6 months if they'd been sent regular, supportive text messages—at first, five times a day, then three times a week.[13] During Stage 1, ask a friend to text you at random times to remind you to write down how you feel, what you've eaten, and how much you have (or have not) been craving your False Fix. Ask your friend to send you messages that emphasize the benefits of the healthy habits you're building, remind you to focus on your successes, and encourage you not to give up just because you had a momentary lapse—all those types of messages were proven most effective. If this works for you, ask your pal to up your "dose": University of Oregon researchers found text message prompts to note craving levels, sent eight times a day for 3 weeks, helped smokers stick to their abstinence program.[14, 15]

Maybe texting's not your thing. No problem! Just apply the same approach to snail mail (yes, people still write cards and letters), Twitter, e-mail, Facebook, instant messaging, Skype, phone calls, or whatever other communication format you favor. (Bonus: Studies show that our dopamine system loves the "ping!" of an unexpected text or e-mail.) In the British study, smokers who asked for more help when they were really stressed did better as well. Pick up the phone or send out a virtual SOS when chips and dip are calling your name— a supportive reply makes a huge (sometimes lifesaving) difference. There are plenty of new apps out there that enable you to program your smartphone or tablet to receive daily pings of motivation and encouragement. (See Appendix F for some of my recommendations.)

Fight back against the lies! You're going to look your inner addict straight in the eye and take control. Listen to the typical seductive whispers in your head:

"Oh, come on, it's *just* a cookie."

"Hey, *just* take one chocolate."

"I'm stressed out of my mind, and I *just* need my fix and I'll be just fine."

"Grow up, it's *just* chips and dip, not heroin or something."

Notice that "just" appears in every phrase? Your brain is trying to convince you that what you're about to do is no big deal. Your inner addict is trying to convince you that consuming that bag or box or tray of False Fixes is not at all like doing a line of cocaine or shooting up with heroin or drinking a gallon of wine. Well, you know by now that science has clearly shown this is a lie. So when you hear any of those phrases, here's what to do:

1. Take a deep breath and with all of your might shout out, "It's a lie!" (If you're in a public place, use it as an internal mantra: "It's a lie, it's a lie, it's a lie.")

2. Keep saying it until you've drummed out the voices in your head.

3. Walk away from the False Fix. Run if you have to. Get out of there.

4. Take another breath and smile. You won this time. Be vigilant.

Stay cool. As you go through your day, when you are given any choice—to meditate, eat well, move more—ask yourself, "Who is in control and whose behavior is this—mine or my inner addict's?" As you progress through Detox, you'll be acutely aware of the tug-of-war between the two until, through perseverance, persistence, patience, and practice, you triumph. The whisper will become barely audible. It will never totally disappear, but your own voice will be the new roaring powerhouse that controls your actions.

Our biggest enemy is the voice in our head that tries to convince us our False Fixes are, in fact, the best thing *ever* and we are *totally missing out* if we don't eat that *delicious, crunchy, satisfying* platter of nachos. Researchers call this a "hot system"—when we focus on the immediate pleasure, and damn the consequences—versus a "cold system," that considers the longer-term implications for making that choice. Use this hot/cold system to your advantage. In one study, some kids were told marshmallows "look like white clouds." Other kids were told marshmallows "look yummy!" Which kids were able to resist the marshmallows better, do you think?[16]

Block your False Fix's reinforcement power. In my previous book *Body-for-Life for Women*, I talked about my dinner with Sharon Stone, during which she sampled a bite from each dessert on the table. When the waiter did not clear the dessert dishes immediately, Sharon promptly poured salt all over them. Perfect example of creating an aversive cue—she interrupted the cycle and took away the False Fix's reinforcement power.

A great trick is to start mentally associating your False Fix with something negative and toxic. Think of the worst experience you ever had after a False Fix binge. Get a red-hot visual of waking up in a bed filled with wrappers and crumbs in the sheets. Burn that memory into your mind. Like a pop-up on your computer, call upon that image every time the False Fix lies start filling your head. This aversive therapy will flip your old addictive motivation-learning-memory reward circuitry on its head.

Take a page from *Sex and the City*'s Miranda, when—after she found herself pulling brownies out of the garbage (and declaring her need to check into the "Betty Crocker Clinic")—she poured dish soap all over the platter of brownies. Heap on the coffee grounds or eggshells or mud if it works. My patient Marlyn created a fabulous aversive cue. While she was in the process of losing 60 pounds, she helped mute the False Fix lies by taking a belt she wore when she was her heaviest, coiling it, and placing it in her fridge front and center. "It sat there for months as a daily reminder of my worst memories of embarrassment, wearing clothes that could fit a family of 12. It was a humble reminder that should I drop my vigilance, my inner addict was just waiting for me to cave." Take a moment and create your own aversive False Fix memories and cues. To fight your addiction, you need to do whatever it takes—this is war!

Create a Healthy Hunger visual reminder. When *The Biggest Loser's* Tara Costa was training for the Ironman triathlon, she created a wristband that said "KONA" and put it on her dominant hand. Whenever she reached for cookies or an extra serving of dinner, she'd see the reminder and think: *Will this cookie/extra serving/ice cream help me be an Ironman? If not, why am I even thinking about it?* Her typical False Fix reward paled in comparison to the joy, excitement, and pride she anticipated upon finishing the Ironman. Put a small reminder of your Healthy Hunger somewhere on your person so you can see it everywhere you go. In the midst of days when you have tsunamis of stress coming at you from every direction, a constant and gentle reminder of why you want to Detox and finally recover from your overeating can be a lifesaver.

Switch fat talk for self-compassion. Imagine you are running a marathon. You are at the 25th mile marker, with a little over 1 mile to go until you cross the finish line and achieve your amazing goal. You spot a friend on the side of the road, waving at you. You swerve over to give her a high five and she yells out, "You'll never make it! What makes you think you can do this? You're kidding yourself. You don't have it in you. You're a loser and you'll never make it."

Totally ludicrous, right? But this is the kind of self-talk we pollute our brains with *every day*. Think of the internal dialogue that flows through your head on a daily basis: "You look horrible in this." "You have no control, you're a fat slob."

What about this commentary is helpful? Nothing. And it's the worst kind of self-speak while you're detoxing. But when you've had this automatic fat talk habit for so long, you can cling to mistaken beliefs that poison your brain. To successfully detox and recover from your False Fixes, you need to develop a new skill: self-compassion.

Self-compassion is the ability to be kind and understanding to yourself when you're suffering or when you feel inadequate in some way. Self-compassion helps you key into your shared humanity, allowing you to see that pain and failure are natural, unavoidable parts of being a human being. Unlike dissociation, self-compassion is not about running away from your feelings—it's about facing them honestly, without resorting to self-pity or turning into a drama queen or king. You will gift yourself with unconditional love and compassion. This is one of the most powerful weapons against the continued attack of False Fixes.

When you don't practice self-compassion, you are more critical of yourself, more apt to seek perfection and be angrier and competitive with others. You're more likely to judge yourself solely on external, changing metrics. Your scale and size rule you. Your whole self-worth is unstable.

On the other hand, self-compassion is about treating yourself with the same respect, honor, loyalty, trust, and love you bestow on your family and friends.

Here are a few shifts from self-critical to self-compassionate:

"I'm stupid." → "Oh well, mistakes happen. Let me try again."

"I suck at this." → "I'm just learning—I'm a work in progress."

"I can't believe I let myself go again." → "No one is perfect—I am human. Now I'm making another choice."

"I look like a fat pig at the gym." → "I'm starting my journey here and will simply do my best, make some friends, and be patient because I know I can do this."

"I feel like such a large, lumpy, undisciplined loser." → "I really enjoy feeding my body this nourishing food."

"This is so horrible—I'll never live through it." → "This is very challenging situation. How can I help myself through this?"

One Wake Forest University study found that when researchers asked young women not to feel bad about eating doughnuts during a taste test ("I hope you won't be hard on yourself—everyone eats unhealthily sometimes"), those participants unconsciously chose to eat less candy later. Those who hadn't been encouraged to be self-compassionate ate more.[17]

Be kind to yourself. It may sound counterintuitive, but kindness and compassion will ultimately lead you to your fittest, healthiest self.

Swim for your island of competence. Most of you probably spend the majority of your time concentrating on what you see as your weaknesses. While it's important to identify places in your life where you are vulnerable to self-destruction, one of the niftiest ways to neutralize any proclaimed weakness is to apply one of your strengths. In order to do that, you need to know what those strengths are.

Define what psychologist Robert Brooks calls the "islands of competence" in your life. What about yourself are you most proud of? What do you love about yourself? Take out a sheet of paper and write every single thing that you love (or even just like) about yourself. If you're unsure, ask some folks you trust, and who really know you, to share with you their perceptions of your strengths. I'll bet you'll be pleasantly surprised!

This is no time for humility, people! Zero modesty! Get it all out there, a full inventory of your awesomeness. No less than 25 things—no matter how small! Feel free to reach to 100, if you can.

Now, take the top five things on this list, the ones you are most proud of, like "I am great at my job" or "I'm really organized" or "My family trusts me" or "I am very kind to strangers and people who need help" or "I stick up for people who are being bullied" or even "I am committed to making the Hunger Fix plan work!" When you feel yourself sinking into fat talk, swim to one of these islands of competence and reach for the hand of your own positive marathon cheerleader. Let her pull you out of the muck with a reminder: "You are not a failure—you are strong, kind, and generous person. And you're kicking butt!"

You can even print this list and tack it somewhere you'll see it every day as a Healthy Hunger visual. Rudyard Kipling said it best: "Words are the most powerful drug used by mankind." Make yours positive, inspiring, Healthy Fixes, and use your words wisely!

Take one day at a time. This adage is an addiction-recovery classic, for a very good reason. *The rest of your life* is overwhelming; *the next 24 hours*, less so. Start every day with a 24-hour commitment: "Today I will _____." Identify one easy-to-execute action that will help you achieve your goal from Mind, Mouth, or Muscle—but just one! Don't go to that extreme place of wanting to be rid of every False Fix *right now*. That impatience and impulsiveness is part of what got you into this mess.

During Detox, when you're still getting used to your new Healthy Fixes lifestyle, you might want to divide your waking hours into two, three, or four segments. Say you're awake for 16 hours. Divide those waking hours into four 4-hour segments. Let's say that your easiest segments are morning and lunch. Okay, you'll whip through those. The struggle begins during the last two segments of the day, because you typically cave to your cravings when you're tired and feeling overwhelmed by midafternoon. This is when you need to crank up your focus and vigilance and have a plan of attack. Make sure you that have your midafternoon snack ready and your dinner planned and that you hit the sack on time so you're not trolling the kitchen looking for something to eat. Most of my patients break up the day into "easy to survive" and "battle zone" segments so that they can zero in on where the hard-core behavioral changes have to happen.

At the end of your 24 hours, look at your schedule and see if you met your goals. If you did, say it out loud to yourself: "I really did well today. I achieved everything I set out to do." If you didn't, do not dissolve into negative self-speak once again. Instead, *look for the lesson*. How can you apply that newfound wisdom tomorrow?

You may plan for the next day: getting the right foods, laying out walking clothes, planning where to be for a meeting. Especially during Detox, but even into Recovery, you are not to look beyond successfully living your life for 24 hours.

Review your EpiphaME. People unsure of their EpiphaME can flounder in the face of temptation. When you depend 100 percent on willpower, your mental reserve can get sapped quickly—leaving you vulnerable to relapse.

Keep your EpiphaME top of mind with this writing exercise. Go back to your day 1 journal—your video or your writing. Listen to yourself. Read your words. Look at your initial photos. Remind yourself why this Detox journey is so important, how it will save your life.

Then do this exercise: For 3 nights in a row, video for 5 minutes and/or write for 15 minutes about what your life will be like when you achieve your EpiphaME. You had an EpiphaME for a reason. It showed you what you really hunger for in your life. See it, feel it, and taste the triumph and victory when you achieve it.

Drill down for details:

- What will your body feel like in your new skinny jeans?
- What will it feel like to run up the stairs or to jump on the trampoline with your kids (or grandkids)?

- What will it feel like to run into old friends and have them not recognize you because you've lost so much weight?
- What will it feel like to not be at the will of your False Fixes?

If you find this exercise helpful, repeat it every week, and constantly create new details: Write and/or video about what a day will look like, what excitement and challenge your new promotion will bring to you, how much fun it will be to pick out smaller clothes for your new adventure. This exercise will help you get through those inevitable tough times.

Find your Hunger Fix tribe. As you progress through your Hunger Fix program, you may need to take a closer look at the people you spend time with. Many members of your current "tribe" may not support or understand your Healthy Fix lifestyle—or they may even try to interfere.

There are three distinct tribes you need to know about.

- **Your enablers.** The first are the people who, deliberately or not, actually encourage your False Fix habits. You need to eliminate these folks, or if that's not possible, minimize your exposure to them. This is a tough one for lots of people, as this group may include friends, family members, and co-workers. Take time to really think this through and observe who "gets it." Sabotage can be subtle: Your friend buys you a margarita at happy hour (despite your earlier pledge not to drink that night), or your husband brings your favorite chips or ice cream into the house after you've asked him not to. Even seemingly positive comments can sound innocent enough: "Wow, you're looking too thin! Have a nice piece of cake." (Yeah, here's the thing: It's no one's business what you eat or what you look like. Let that PFC of yours kick in and help you scan for enablers.)
- **Your Hunger Fix peers.** The second tribe includes people who are just like you. They have suffered with the same False Fix habits and are at some stage of their own journey to improve themselves. You can identify with them and use them in a mutually beneficial way.

The reason 12-step programs succeed with drug addicts is not necessarily the program itself—it's the other people at the meetings. Positive peer pressure really works. Just keep in mind that you want to hang out with people who are authentically committed to achieve progress in their lives. Avoid folks who've come to a grinding halt in their recovery and who spend most of their time blaming others for their addiction. They need help, but you're not their therapist. Instead, seek out those who, like you, are committed to taking it a day at a time, striving to realize their dream of a life rich with joy and worth living. One study on alcoholics found that a strong social network helps addicts reduce their impulsivity, improve their coping skills, and stick with their program for the long term.[18] When you surround yourself with people you love and respect, they'll remind you why you're doing the Hunger Fix program and keep you motivated to reach your goals.

- **Your Healthy Hunger mentors.** The third tribe is populated by people who care about you but have not been directly afflicted by your False Fix issues. The field of research into social contagion suggests the people you associate with can have a tremendous impact on your health. Essentially, the research says, you can "catch" a positive attitude or less-fattening diet simply from being friends with happier, fitter people. For example, when you morph from sedentary to running, suddenly you're surrounded by other runners who want to support your journey. Your mentor tribe can include your trainer, running buddy, therapist, personal journal, best friend, spouse, and any mentor, plus Internet support groups found through WebMD, SparkPeople, Weight Watchers, Take Off Pounds Sensibly (TOPS), Curves, Overeaters Anonymous Web sites or through Facebook (create your own page). Even your pets—your dog, cat, bird—can be your mentors, showering you with unconditional love and acceptance. And hey, don't forget to include your doctor, particularly if he or she makes you feel accepted and supported in your struggle. No shaming allowed! One study found that diabetic patients of doctors who scored highest on empathy ratings had a 30 percent greater improvement on their hemoglobin A1C and LDL cholesterol tests than patients of doctors with low empathy.[19] The researchers believe the results come down to trust: The more you trust your doctor *really* cares about you, the more likely you are to listen to his or her recommendations.

Find extra time for a joyful belly-laughing high. Laughter activates dopamine release in the midbrain and hypothalamus, producing a rush of pleasure and instantly reinforcing that experience. You'll simultaneously get a burst of relaxing endorphins and metabolism-boosting growth hormone,[20] which also enhances cognition and slows aging. Triple bonus: If your spouse or partner can surprise you and delight your brain to the point of making you crack up, you'll be constantly rewarded—and reinforced—for being with him or her. Make plans that don't revolve around food, or try a new, active hobby together.

Vigilance is victory. One thing you must remember as you embark on your Healthy Fix lifestyle journey: If you stop being vigilant, your addictive habits will subtly, slowly take control. The next thing you know, you're swimming in False Fixes. This doesn't mean you should turn yourself into a basket case of compulsive obsessing about every habit you practice. It simply means that you need to get used to scanning your living environment and being cautious about the addictive cues, triggers, and temptations that you face daily.

When you first learned to drive a car, you clung to the steering wheel, hypervigilant of every nuance in your surroundings—because driving was all new for you. Once you became an experienced driver, you relaxed that death grip on the steering wheel (let's hope!). However, you haven't stopped being vigilant—you just do it in a more relaxed way. The Hunger Fix is exactly the same. Stay aware from this moment on. Get your False Fix radar revved up. That vigilant focus will be your own built-in protector, like safe driving. You'll need it now, tomorrow, and for the rest of your life.

Stage 1: Mouth

Alcoholics and crack addicts have it easy—they can just "say no." You? Not possible. Food addiction is more complex. Most people are addicted to combos—savory/salty/starchy or sweet/fat or fat/starchy. One of the main reasons the Hunger Fix plan works so well is because it sidesteps these combinations and substitutes the False Fix foods with tasty, delicious, and pleasurable Healthy Fix *food* options.

Of the combinations above, sugar/fat is the most potent. But before you breathe a sigh of relief and say, "Oh, I don't have a sweet tooth," remember that any refined carb is actually a sugar. When you think of it that way, it's hard to imagine any False Fix food that doesn't have that sugar/fat combination—pasta with cheese, white bread with butter, chocolate-covered pretzels, cheese pizza, cheeseburger on a sesame seed bun, cheese fries . . . the list is endless.

Many food addicts enter Detox feeling fearful, filled with shame, and in a terrible relationship with food. They're food phobic. Food is what caused this problem. Food is the enemy. Stage 1: Mouth is about reframing and redefining that relationship. I'm here to gently show you how to eat safely, decrease your fear of deprivation by increasing natural rewards, and quiet your addictive urges and impulses.

In Stage 1: Mouth, your primary objective will be to stay the heck away from your most dangerous foods, the False Fix foods that will guarantee that you will lose control. You'll also begin the Hunger Fix eating plan. Check out the meal plan and recipes in Chapters 8 and 9. In Stage 1: Detox, the goal is to experience your own natural "safe high" with foods that increase dopamine and thus the pleasure and reward you seek.

We'll shoot for a nutrient mix of 30 percent lean protein; 30 to 35 percent healthy fat; and 30 to 35 percent carbohydrates, primarily as vegetables, fruit, and whole grain—in other words, percentages with enough protein to keep you sated and enough healthy fats to keep your brain plumped up and growing new neurons and receptors. Modify this nutrient mix as needed with your doctor's guidance.

We'll also shoot for 20 grams of daily soluble fiber. A recent study found that for every 10 grams of increased daily soluble fiber intake, you'll experience a 3.7 percent decrease in accumulation of toxic visceral fat.[21] (If the person also exercised regularly, the decrease was 7.4 percent!) In "food" terms, you could hit (and even exceed) your soluble fiber target by eating the following foods over the course of a day:

- ½ cup oatmeal (3 grams fiber)
- 1 small banana (3 grams)
- ½ cup cooked red or black beans (7 grams)
- 1 small apple (5 grams)
- ½ cup lentils (8 grams)
- ½ cup blueberries (3 grams)

Let's take get started on all the facets of Stage 1: Detox's Mouth plan.

Name your False Fix foods. Take out the food inventory lists you created in Chapter 4. Look at the list of the foods you eat regularly, and find your specific False Fix foods. (I also call these your "bingeables.") These are foods that, once you have consumed a serving, leave you with a feeling of being out of control and result in your reaching for more and overeating every time. They're the foods you sneak eat, the bad boys you score at your favorite grocer or bakery or candy store. You end up in a food coma—and when you snap back to reality, you're filled with negative and defeated emotions. These foods are nothing but trouble. They simply don't work for you and probably never will.

The solution? Never touch them again.

If you have an addictive family background, you may already know what I'm talking about. Here's a common example: Let's say your dad was an alcoholic. Think of the worst experience you ever had with him. Maybe he always stunk of scotch, or he would be mean to your mom when he was drinking, or he was in a few car accidents. Think back to how horrified you were when you saw that and knew that it was from the alcohol.

Now, whenever you see your False Fix in your mind, I want you to start associating it in your mind with the scotch—because that's what you're doing. You're not drinking his scotch, but you are drinking your chocolate. You're shooting it up. You're freebasing it. You're *doing* chocolate.

Once they identify these foods, my patients will often plead, "Well, you know, what if I *just* have a little bit?"

Your dad couldn't have *just* one scotch, and maybe you can't have *just* one cookie—maybe you end up eating three boxes of them. Three thousand calories later, there you sit, blacked out in a food coma, every bit as rock bottom as your dad was when he blacked out after a bender.

Everyone has a drug of choice. Paula Abdul was a binger and a bulimic, and she loved hard-core sugar candy like Red Hots and Good & Plenty. She struggled for two decades until she underwent successful rehab. A patient of mine says most of the foods she abuses are round foods—bagels, doughnuts, cookies, pizza, cakes. Personally, potato chips don't interest me, and I hate salt. But if you put gourmet jelly beans in front of me, watch out. Therefore, I have decided to abstain from this particular False Fix.

Dr. Arya Sharma compares food addicts' need to abstain with another chronic illness: "Recognizing that someone has a hypersensitive bronchial system that predisposes them to asthma should lead them to avoid and eliminate airborne pollutants in their immediate environment—rather than simply try to breathe less."

Your False Fix foods are poisonous to your mind and body. Break free. You are powerful enough to say no.

Build your medicine chest of "safe highs." OK, you've identified the False Fix foods that will activate your addiction and send you into an over eating food frenzy. You write 'em off. No more False Fixes.

But the Hunger Fix plan doesn't just leave you high and dry. the goal throughout the program is to keep you as high as possible—safely, on tasty, rewarding Healthy Fix food options.

Look at your food inventory again and find the healthy foods that are left. These are the nonbingeables that you can live with right now. You obviously like them—they're on your regular list. Check out the calorie counts—they could be an eye-opener as well. You learn that blueberries are 60 calories a cup, so what the heck—eat 3 cups if you want to! You're still much better off than finishing an entire cake.

Now, you'll transition to safe high foods. My patients have found that safe high foods are "freeing" because they decrease the sense of deprivation. Safe highs are characterized by a combination of fiber and protein (with or without a healthy carb or fat). Protein increases satiety and kills the addictive carb craving. Science shows that when you have that fiber and protein combo, the body senses the macronutrients, and the sphincter muscle that leads from the stomach to the small intestine closes to allow the food to rest longer in the stomach, prolonging the breakdown of the protein and fiber. This creates a greater sense of stomach fullness, decreasing appetite as well as hunger.

Safe Highs (pick one from each column)

Fiber		Protein
Berries	+	Cottage cheese
Apple	+	Peanut butter
Celery	+	Almond butter
Wasa crisps	+	Coconut butter
Wheat bran	+	Greek yogurt
Broccoli	+	Low-fat cheese
Carrots	+	Hummus
Peppers	+	Black bean dip
Avocado	+	Vegetarian baked beans

Cut the cravings, ditch the deprivation. You have to keep your body sated and your dopamine levels supported because an addicted brain will read any sign of deprivation as a stress that requires "medication"—in the form of a doughnut or bag of chips. A *Proceedings of the National Academy of Sciences* study found that when rats who'd had access to sugar and chocolate-flavored treats had those treats withheld, the rats' central nucleus of the amygdala released *five times* the normal levels of corticotropin-releasing factor, or CRF, a stress hormone linked to motivation—the same hormone that junkies release while going through withdrawal. The rats were strung out and jittery and didn't want to touch their normal food—they wanted the sugar and chocolate. And when they got those treats, they ate even more than before—and their stress hormones returned to normal levels.[22]

Food deprivation makes False Fixes seem that much more attrac-

I Need a Fix

Eric's Delightful "Safe Highs"

Forty-seven-old Eric thought his DNA was his destiny. The product of a hefty family tree populated by big guys and big guts, 6-foot-1 Eric decided to take himself on when his weight hit 270—along with high blood pressure and cholesterol. A self-described food addict, he'd always felt out of control around any plate of starchy, salty, fatty foods. Sweets were not his thing. A red-meat-and-potatoes, bread-and-pasta kind of man, he wouldn't have known a vegetable if it knocked down his front door.

He confessed that he was worried about feeling hungry and deprived if he left his classic American cuisine. But once he started the Hunger Fix program, he was surprised how satisfying fish, poultry, legumes, and dairy products could be. He ditched the bread and nearly grew chicken feathers and turkey wings from his newfound love for poultry, and he has never been more regular (ahem!) thanks to the heaps of vegetables and Healthy Fix toppings he treats himself to. Eating his new safe high combos, hopping on his elliptical trainer daily, and making time for prayer and meditation helped him pare off 50 pounds.

tive—obviously! It also starts to increase the rewarding effects of other drugs. In other words, the traditional approach to dieting not only sets you up for relapse into rebound weight gain, it also primes your brain to be addicted to even more dangerous False Fixes, such as cocaine or alcohol.[23]

You probably experienced this for years with yo-yo dieting. It's not only about that old "lowered set point/you're hungry-but-body-needs-fewer-calories" thing—it's the fact that your brain is literally going through withdrawal.

This is why diets are never the answer and a major reason why they fail, big-time. We are steering clear of that yo-yo dieting mind-set. In Stage 1, you change the foods that you eat—but you do not touch the quantities. You can have as many whole foods—low-calorie, nutrient-rich vegetables, fruits, lean meats, beans, and low-fat dairy (milk, yogurt, cheese)—as you want. Enjoy the taste and reward while feeling full and satisfied. Cravings, *what* cravings? Let loose on produce. As you progress from Detox to Recovery, we'll continue to refine this issue of how much you eat. For now, dig into your veggies, protein, and berries.

But this whole foods bonanza has one notable exception: Grains must be tightly limited. Stick to single servings of whole grains only—quinoa, barley, brown rice. Grains can easily become False Fixes when you're trying to Detox from other carb-based fixes. If grains become a problem, you eliminate them for now.

Use your cross-addictions. When people successfully kick addictions such as alcohol, drugs or cigarettes, gambling, or sex addiction, they have trained their brains to simply say, "That _____ does not and will never work for me." The good news is, if you've had this experience, you have a head start on the Hunger Fix—you'll be better able to identify the signals of which addictive foods will lead you to danger. Double down on that identification; start visualizing/perceiving them like the alcohol, drugs, or cigs you have already successfully rejected.

Keep a tight rein on the five W's.

Who: Are your dining companions False Fix enablers, or do they support your desire to choose Healthy Fixes instead?

What: Follow the Hunger Fix plan in Chapter 8, but if you must move off of your program, stick with safe highs or Detox-to-Recovery Transition Foods (see opposite).

When: Are you eating every 3 to 4 hours to maintain excellent blood sugar levels and to keep appetite and cravings under control? Are you avoiding old patterns, like omitting those important mid-afternoon snacks, skipping lunch, or, worse, eating late at night?

Where: Are you eating while sitting at a table in a kitchen or dining room? (In other words, are you grazing over your computer all day or mindlessly chowing down in bed, watching a *Law & Order* marathon.)

Why: Why are you sneaking a snack? Try to remember HALT: Am I hungry, angry, lonely, or tired? What's the emotion triggering the False Fix? Or is it the buzz from the three glasses of wine you just had that's telling you it's okay to order hot wings?

Detox-to-Recovery Transition Foods. Sometimes, when we think about giving up our False Fixes, we get all emotional: "Do I really have to give it up? Will I never get to have it again?" I can't tell you that—only you can decide what belongs on your False Fix list. But perhaps these transition foods can help.

Foods in the far left column raise dopamine—but they are also high in the type of sugar, salt, and/or fats that have the power to alter reward pathways in the brain. Baby-step your way from those False Fixes over to the right-hand column of Healthy Fix all-stars.

(One caveat: Diet soda is used frequently by folks detoxing, but it should not be used forever. Artificial sweeteners like aspartame, saccharine, or Splenda can increase appetite and increase cravings for sweets, perpetuating the False Fix. Treat diet soda like a nicotine patch—use it only for a limited time, to get off sugar soda.)

Become a gum junkie. Long a staple of recovering addicts, gum can

Detox-to-Recovery Transition Foods

False Fix (Pre-Detox)	Less False Fix (Stage 1)	More Healthy Fix (Stage 2)	Most Healthy Fix (Stage 3)
Sugar soda	Diet soda	Seltzer water	Still water
Bacon cheeseburger	Lean beef burger	Turkey burger	Bean burger
Iceberg with creamy dressing	Romaine with creamy dressing	Romaine with balsamic vinaigrette	Spinach with balsamic vinaigrette
Fast-food fries	Homemade baked fries	Homemade sweet potato fries	Roasted sweet potatoes
Full-fat potato chips	Air-popped popcorn	Carrot sticks	Kale chips

help you tame the food addiction beast for a variety of reasons. First, of course, it puts a foodlike substance in your mouth and gives your jaws something to do instead of mow through chips. When you chew gum, you cause a repetitive movement, which spurs the brain to release more serotonin. The large chewing muscles have a huge venous plexus that warms up and immediately warms the anterior hypothalamus, resulting in yet more serotonin. You can chew your way through Detox (and get some toned facial muscles while you're at it)—it's a quick and private way to calm yourself in any situation. Look for gum sweetened with xylitol; this naturally occurring sugar substitute has been found to reduce cavities.[24] Animal studies suggest it may even help prevent insulin resistance and belly fat accumulation.[25]

Construct your diet around dopamine-building foods. Recently, researchers at the McKnight Brain Institute at the University of Florida suggested a novel line of treatment for addiction, called deprivation-amplification relapse therapy (or DART). Part of this revolutionary program suggests that increasing dopamine with the amino acids tyrosine and phenylalanine can help relieve the ease the transition off False Fixes.

The resulting increased levels of dopamine can help to satisfy the especially sensitive D2 receptors that might be itching for more dopamine—an urge that, if not satisfied, can often lead to relapse.[26]

Below are dopamine-building nutrients and foods you can add to your diet.

Phenylalanine is essential—meaning your body can only get it from foods you eat. When people don't have enough phenylalanine in their diet, they can feel confused, lack energy, and suffer from depression, decreased alertness, and memory problems.[27]

Foods High in Phenylalanine[28]

Meat and Eggs	Cured ham, top round beef, New Zealand lamb, turkey legs, veal, top loin pork bottom round, stewed chicken, beef brisket, pork loin, pot roast, broiled chicken, top sirloin, goat meat, pastrami, turkey breast, rib eye, pork tenderloin, pheasant, emu, ostrich, dark meat turkey, rabbit, bison, chicken drumsticks, bottom sirloin, mutton, goose, duck, ground 95% lean beef, guinea hen, turkey ham, turkey pastrami, eggs
Fish and Seafood	Catfish, rainbow trout, salmon, octopus, tilefish, freshwater bass, striped mullet, swordfish, bluefin tuna, dried whitefish, yellowtail, clams, squid, anchovies, surimi, shrimp, sturgeon, gefilte fish, albalone, mackerel, light canned tuna, white canned tuna, blue crab, canned pink salmon, trout, dried and salted cod, shellfish
Dairy	Milk (fat-free, 1%, or 2%), cottage cheese, plain fat-free yogurt, shredded Parmesan cheese
Vegetables	Frozen spinach, fresh boiled spinach, raw spinach, canned turnip greens, raw broccoli rabe, Swiss chard, fresh basil, amaranth leaves
Fruits	Watermelon
Nuts and Seeds	Watermelon seeds, fenugreek, roasted soybean nuts, lupin seeds
Legumes and Beans	Firm and soft tofu, soybean protein, soybean flour, pigeon peas
Extras	Chocolate, drinks or gum containing aspartame (Equal), baker's yeast, soy sauce

Tyrosine is a nonessential amino acid, because your body can make it from phenylalanine. But if you eat foods with tyrosine, the path is more direct—as soon as it's in your bloodstream, it gets transported into the brain and converted into dopamine to be stored up for release.[29] Tyrosine is also involved in the production of thyroid hormones, as well as the stress hormones epinephrine and norepinephrine. During times of stress, tyrosine may be drawn away from dopamine production in favor of these hormones, and your body may not make enough tyrosine from phenylalanine. That's why, in your daily diet, but especially during times of stress, tyrosine-rich foods may help protect your dopamine supply.[30]

Foods High in Tyrosine[31]

Meat and Eggs	Chicken, turkey, pork, eggs, egg whites, buffalo, shrimp, moose, elk, pork loin, duck, rabbit, venison, ostrich, pheasant, Cornish game hen, beef brisket, pot roast, 95% lean ground beef, bison
Fish and Seafood	Salmon, caviar, orange roughy, light canned tuna, Pacific cod, sunfish, dolphin fish, Atlantic cod, haddock, yellowfin tuna, Alaska king crab, skipjack tuna, perch, pollock, pike, tilapia, flounder, sole, lobster, walleye pike, snapper, crayfish, blue crab, Dungeness crab, Pacific rockfish, halibut, monkfish, sea bass, striped bass, scallop, sturgeon, clam, swordfish, shark, squid, anchovies, carp
Dairy	Milk (fat-free, 1%, or 2%), cheese, yogurt, cottage cheese, fat-free cream cheese, low-fat cheddar or Colby cheese, fresh Parmesan cheese, low-fat provolone cheese, part-skim mozzarella, dried milk, evaporated fat-free milk, romano cheese
Vegetables	Spirulina, pumpkin leaves, mustard greens, frozen spinach, boiled spinach, watercress, horseradish, raw spinach, canned spinach, turnip greens
Fruits	Avocados, bananas
Nuts and Seeds	Almonds, sesame seeds, pumpkin seeds
Legumes and Beans	Soy products, soy protein isolate, soy protein concentrate, peanuts, kidney beans, peanut flour, firm tofu, soy flour, lima beans
Whole Grains	Whole wheat, steel-cut oats

Vitamin B$_6$ forms the coenzyme necessary to convert these amino acids into dopamine and norepinephrine.[32] A diet stocked with tyrosine- and phenylalanine-building foods can get a little protein heavy. Many meats (such as salmon, chicken, and turkey) have both. But luckily, vitamin B$_6$ is also found in many fruits and vegetables, which should form the foundation of your Hunger Fix eating plan and which will help you get antioxidants and other essential nutrients that help your body heal, prevent cravings, and build new brain matter.

Many of these foods are high in soluble fiber, which helps to balance your blood sugar and reduce visceral fat, and insoluble fiber, which, when combined with the protein, helps trigger that stomach sphincter reflex that keeps you fuller longer.

Foods High in Vitamin B$_6$

Meat and Eggs	Turkey, chicken, calf's liver, beef tenderloin, venison
Fish and Seafood	Yellowfin tuna, salmon, cod, snapper, halibut
Vegetables	Russet potatoes, spinach, red bell peppers, turnip greens, garlic, cauliflower, mustard greens, celery, cabbage, crimini mushrooms, asparagus, broccoli, kale, collard greens, brussels sprouts, Swiss chard, leeks, tomato, carrots, summer squash, eggplant, romaine lettuce, onions, sweet potato, green beans, yam, winter squash
Fruits	Bananas, watermelon, cantaloupe, strawberries, avocados, pineapple, grapes
Nuts and Seeds	Hazelnuts, flaxseeds
Legumes and Beans	Soy protein isolate, soyburger, lentils, garbanzo beans (chickpeas), pink beans, lima beans, pinto beans, peanut flour, peanuts, great Northern beans, yellow beans, small white beans, navy beans, pink lentils, tofu, black beans, pigeon peas
Whole Grains	Fortified cereals, brown rice, wheat germ
Spices and Extras	Garlic, cayenne pepper, tumeric, blackstrap molasses, ginger

No restaurants for Stage 1. Because the portion sizes are so out of control at many restaurants these days—and the healthy choices are so scant—I'm banning restaurants for you during Stage 1. A National Institutes of Health study found that women, whether they're dieting or binge eaters, tend to consume way more fat and calories on the days they eat in restaurants. In fact, about 30 percent of all binges happen in restaurants. The researchers called restaurants "high risk food environments"—definitely not for you during Detox.[33] Does a recovering alcoholic hang out in bars? Absolutely not.

Of course, I know that it may be difficult for some of you to avoid restaurants due to your work and lifestyle. I'm just advocating that, whenever possible, steer clear to stay safe. However, should you absolutely have to eat out, find restaurants where your meals can model those in the Stage 1 meal plan (which starts on page 223).

Limit sugars. We've talked about how crazy-addictive sugars can be. Refined and processed sugars awaken the sleeping dragon of addiction in susceptible people. Even if you're not addicted, sugars will increase your insulin levels and cause a blood sugar crash—resulting in an insatiable appetite for more. And though the combination of "layered" sugar and fat has less of an insulin punch, it triggers a higher opioid response—Dr. David Kessler termed this combination "hyperpalatable" in his book *The End of Overeating.*

To bring down your daily added sugar intake, you will need to read food ingredient labels carefully. One gram of sugar contains 4 calories, so any innocent-looking tasty morsel with 20 grams of sugar will instantly add 80 calories to that serving, on top of all the other ingredients. One 12-ounce can of regular soda contains 8 teaspoons of sugar— or 130 empty calories (meaning calories with no nutritional value). According to the American Heart Association, women should consume no more than 100 calories from added sugars per day, and men 150 calories per day. Science also shows that by cutting carbs in total, you can increase the efficiency of the fat-burning metabolism in the body.

Continue to look carefully at the list of ingredients for added sugars (which may be included under several names, many ending with the letters *ose*, such as sucrose, maltose, etc.), as well as high fructose corn syrup, molasses, cane sugar, corn sweetener, raw sugar, syrup, honey, or fruit juice concentrates.

Ban trans fats. A Spanish study conducted on over 12,000 people for 6 years found that those who ate a lot of trans fats had a 48 percent higher risk of depression—and, in a dose-response relationship, the more trans fats they ate, the more depressed they became. And this study was done in a country where trans fats make up only 0.4 percent of the total diet. What would that mean in the United States, where trans fats make up 2.5 percent?[34] Check your labels and steer clear.

High Fructose Corn Syrup

I know in a few years we'll look back on high fructose corn syrup and say, "What were we thinking?" A recent study published in the journal *Diabetes, Obesity and Metabolism* used fMRI scans to watch what happens to the brain as people ate fructose or glucose. There was no difference in the way the appetite center of the brain in the hypothalamus reacted to both—but there was a huge difference in the way the cortical control areas responded. With glucose, these areas responsible for how we respond to taste, smells, and visual images clearly reacted the more glucose was administered. By contrast, the fructose did not activate the brain at all—it was as neutral as saline, the control substance. Researchers supposed this might help us to piece together the mystery of why high levels of fructose in the diet seems to correlate with overeating.[35]

The *New York Times* reported on a series of primate experiments that are being done to determine the root causes of obesity. Interestingly, these studies have found that primates given access to high-fat chow don't actually begin to gain excessive weight until they start drinking a fruit punch with high fructose corn syrup—in an amount that's about equivalent to a human drinking one can of soda per day. Then they start to consume about twice as many calories as a normal-weight monkey. The researchers at the Southwest National Primate Research Center in San Antonio said that the addition of the HFCS to the primates' diet seems to put the pedal to the medal toward obesity and diabetes in a way that other foods simply do not.[36]

Stage 1: Muscle

Exercise is the best Healthy Fix because it directly regenerates D2-like dopamine receptors—similar to those linked with food addiction—in the brain, helping to rebuild the brain from the damage of past addiction and prevent it in the future.[37] And it doesn't require a gym membership or an elliptical trainer or a set of barbells. It simply means moving your body. As little as a 5-minute walk around the block or 30 jumping jacks has been shown to reduce the intensity of withdrawal symptoms.[38]

One Vanderbilt University study found that ten 30-minute sessions of moderate treadmill walking over 2 weeks was enough to cut joint smoking by addicted potheads in half, even though they weren't asked to cut down and had, in fact, explicitly said they didn't want to. Even after the study was over, they still cut their original intake by a third.

Researchers believe that the exercise altered the reward circuits in the brain to the point where the exercise took the place of the cannabis—and the exercise started to become self-reinforcing, leading the addicts to need less pot to get the same high. The exercise also decreased their cravings, compulsiveness, emotional ups and downs, and their desperate focus on weed.[39]

I ask you: If exercise can help people who don't even *want* to quit, how much could it help you—someone who's armed and ready to make a huge change?

Take it easy. When I say *exercise*, I want to be clear that you don't have to slap on the Lycra and join a road race—unless you're really ready for that. In fact, I want you to start small and slow. Not only will lowering expectations make it easier for you to get out the door, moderate exercise is actually better for your recovering brain.

Studies on marathoners have found that very vigorous exercise increases the appetite partly because it depresses the amount of the essential nutrient choline, a precursor to the neurotransmitter acetylcholine, by 40 percent.[40] Acetylcholine factors into memory and energy levels, and recent research suggests it also factors in the "rebound" effect some addicts face when they're tempted into a brief relapse.[41] Sometimes False Fixes like smoking create extra acetylcholine receptors in the brain, and when you take away the drug stimulus, those receptors are left wanting.

Combine this all together, and you can see that extreme exercise depletes acetylcholine levels at exactly the time you need them most. In contrast, moderate exercise helps preserve your choline and acetylcholine levels while it increases dopamine. Scores of research studies have shown that a simple practice like walking 30 minutes encourages the consistency that's sustainable for a lifetime. In Stage 3, you may choose to move on to more challenging physical goals—but even if you don't, this moderate, consistent approach will serve you well forever.

Use repetitive movements. Aerobic exercise stimulates parts of your brain that secrete serotonin, which calms you down. But when you do physical movement repetitively, like walking, inline skating, swimming, or climbing on the stair-stepper, those repetitive movements warm your blood to such a degree that when that blood hits the anterior hypothalamus in your brain, *more* serotonin is secreted. Other options include light hiking, elliptical training, treadmill walk-jog mix, NordicTrack, cycling, or even a stationary bike. This rhythmic exercise is like taking an extra "hit" of your mellow drug. Better living through your own chemistry!

Big step, Big Brain. To enjoy the greatest weight-management and maintenance reward, you need to integrate some cardio into your daily life. But no zombie-walking. Inject vitality into every step you take. You'll customize this cardio to your own unique physical needs. If you have any physical disability, please work with the guidance of your medical/rehab/fitness team to find an enjoyable, beneficial activity.

Most studies have found that walking is king. Indeed, one randomized controlled fMRI study published in the *Proceedings of the National Academy of Sciences* found that after a year of taking 40-minute walks three times a week, sedentary older adults grew their hippocampi by 2 percent—reversing their brains' aging process by almost 2 years. This versus those who remained sedentary, whose brains *shrunk* by almost the same amount.[42] (Two more great years for just three walks a week? What a deal—I'll take it!)

Before beginning any activity routine, you need to assess your current physical status and gradually increase your frequency and intensity.

Take adult recess. Instead of thinking of exercise as something "healthy"—which, at the beginning of the program, may seem synonymous with "boring"—think of it as "adult recess" throughout the day. Put on your iPod or crank up the radio and dance to your favorite songs for 10 minutes. In the privacy of your home, let loose and dance like mad! How about some of that amazing Zumba music? Get up and dance like mad. Do it barefoot, naked, who cares? Having fun builds happy genes, rewards you by killing cravings and boosts your energy and immune system. If you feel self-conscious even on your own, you can simply run little steps in place.

Stick with it. Lab rats who'd exercised for 6 weeks reduced their sensitivity to the effects of cocaine—they could have it as much as they wanted, but they voluntarily opted for less cocaine, and to consume it less often, than the rats who'd been sitting around the whole time.[43] Repeated regular exercise triggers the production of enzymes that create receptors in the reward center of your brain. With every step, hop, or dance move you make, you are rebuilding your damaged reward system on a cellular, neurochemical, and habitual level.

Sex it up! With a partner, or even on your own! Sex is not only a huge source of dopamine, it's also a tremendously potent neurogenesis machine in the hippocampus. Long after you and your partner have settled into a cozy sex routine, the act of getting it on will still be producing new brain cells and stimulating the growth of dendritic spines while it acts as a powerful antianxiety agent. Bonus: Women who work out more often have more frequent, faster, and more intense orgasms. This is your brain on sex![44]

Sleep tight. Lack of sleep makes everything harder, and that includes the decision making that your PFC engages in countless times a day.

Researchers from Singapore and the United States reported that when volunteers were sleep deprived, the neural signals reaching their PFC were altered compared to when they were rested (as shown by MRI brain scans). The changes correlated with changes in the study participants' preferences for rewards during a computer game. How the lack of sleep affected the participants varied widely: Some became more willing to hold on to the points they scored in the game for a bigger reward; others were more prone to spending their points for an immediate reward. But the study makes it clear, as the researchers pointed out, that we can't assume we'll make the same value judgments when we're sleep deprived that we would when we're well rested.[45]

A Note to Food Addicts of Average Weight

Earlier on, we mentioned that food addiction is not solely the domain of the overweight and obese. Plenty of men and women appear quite slim and trim but harbor a little secret—they live every day with the torment and struggle of food addiction. They've just learned to control any weight gain by overexercising and/or restricting their calories to make up for relapses and binges. One woman confessed to me that, at size 6 and looking healthy, all she ate every day was junk—just small quantities of junk. She felt rotten and unhealthy and locked in a nightmare of endless cravings for her False Fixes.

To all of you who share her experience, the Healthy Fix lifestyle can help free you from this never-ending torture chamber of out-of-control False Hunger. Many of you are actually "skinny fat" people—you are of average weight, but due to funky eating habits and either no exercise or too much, you've lost lots of muscle and therefore, relatively speaking, you carry too much body fat. You should also find a Clothes-O-Meter to help you gauge the differences in your body throughout Detox, although your changes may be more modest than those who have more pounds to lose. But your Stage 2 measurement targets will be less about body weight than about reaching a normal body fat range for your age. See Appendix E for ranges.

The most important reward is to finally Detox off the False Fixes and onto the Healthy Fixes. You'll be switching your brain's motivation-learning-memory reward circuitry to control your food addiction for life.

If it's lack of sleep that's sapping your willpower, a good first step toward restfulness is to evaluate and work on your sleep hygiene. We're not talking about keeping your blankets clean and washed here (though that's obviously important!). Sleep hygiene means practicing all the habits that prime your body for a good night's sleep and jettisoning the ones that will keep you awake:

- Start by establishing a nightly routine that will get you in bed at roughly the same time every night, and set your alarm to wake you up at the same time every morning (yes, including the weekend).

- In the hours before bedtime, avoid heavy exercise, caffeine, alcohol, and anything that will get your brain spinning.

- Cut off all TV and computer time before bed, too.

- A warm bath before bed will trigger your body to cool down afterward, hastening sleep.

- Make sure your bedroom is dark and quiet.

- And reserve your bed for sleep (and sex) only . . . no watching TV, working on your laptop, snacking, or anything else. This will train your body to associate the bed with sleep.

Slipping and Sliding Toward Recovery

By nature, the learning process is fraught with endless trial and error, experimentation, and self-discovery. Expect to make mistakes and do a little slippin' and slidin' as you go along. This is normal, people! How does a child learn to walk? By hitting the deck a thousand times until she gets it with staying vertical.

Your genes need time to adapt to your new lifestyle, rewarding you with a stronger PFC, more brain cells to combat cravings, and a powerful focus to keep you on track. Look at each choice through the lens of "What's in it for me?" Your ever-growing brain will start to see right through the lie of the False Fix, even in the most stressful of circumstances.

CHAPTER 6

Stage 2: Beginner Recovery

THAT WHICH WE PERSIST IN DOING BECOMES EASIER—
NOT THAT THE NATURE OF THE TASK HAS CHANGED,
BUT OUR ABILITY TO DO HAS INCREASED.
—RALPH WALDO EMERSON

Length of Time: Whatever time it takes to achieve at least 80 percent of the Hunger Fix weight loss/goal/reward + 6 months

Beginner Recovery Reward: Achieve at least 80 percent of the Hunger Fix weight-removal goal, improve body composition, and maintain or continue to refine for 6 months (see Appendix E to determine a healthy range); reduce body fat percentage (doesn't matter how much—any reduction means your body composition is improving); fit into and continue to drop your Clothes-O-Meter sizes; improve physical fitness; become more stress resilient; increase mental energy; become calmer and more centered.

STOP FOR A MOMENT, SIT SOMEWHERE COMFORTABLE, and take a long, deep, cleansing breath. Now pat yourself on the back. Whatever it took and however long you worked at it, you achieved your reward and are transitioning from Stage 1: Detox to your beginner's recovery in Stage 2.

I bet you are filled with a mix of excitement ("Wow, look at me! I am kicking butt here!") and trepidation ("I've been down this road before and have always blown it"). That's okay. Your feelings are completely normal. But let's look at why you have this fear of failure.

When you've endured a long period of food addiction, you've likely had this experience: You're really "good" on a "diet" for a while, and then you're placed in a stressful situation—you have a crushing work deadline or your mom goes into the hospital or you and your partner have a big blowup. Kaboom, your stress hormone levels hit the ceiling, you're blinded by anxiety, and then the three horsemen of the apocalypse show up: helplessness, hopelessness, and defeat.

You cave. You seek shelter with your False Fix. And then, *wham*. The flavors are way more intense than you remember. Sweets are really sweet, fats are even more tempting, and you cannot get enough of your salty starches. You think to yourself, "This is amazing. Seriously, I think this is the best thing I've ever had in my life. Man, my fix never tasted so good."

Then one piece of chocolate becomes four bars. One cookie becomes two boxes. You scarf up the whole pizza.

How is that so?

We now know that when you awaken the sleeping dragon of addiction, it becomes stronger, more powerful, and twice as deadly as before. This effect is exactly the same thing that causes so many relapses on *Celebrity Rehab*. Our hearts break when we witness the drug and alcohol overdoses that occur just months after the stars leave Dr. Drew's care. It wasn't because the celebrities are "weak" or "bad"—any more than your intensely enjoyable reacquaintance with chocolate makes you weak. It's due to a specific biological phenomenon called "supersensitivity." When an addicted person is deprived of her fix, her drug of choice, for a while, and then she encounters it again, the dopamine rush that results is that much more powerful— exactly *because* that person is recuperating.

You see, an addict's dopamine receptors have started to rebound during that downtime—in traditional rehab, receptors can replenish by upward of 20 to 40 percent. The addict's brain is developing the ability to feel pleasure again. If he should get a "hit" of his drug during this supersensitive time, the partially rehabilitated brain's increased receptors draw that much more pleasure out of it. The former addict doesn't have a high tolerance anymore. And the addiction rears its head and says, "Oh my God, this is even better than I thought it was—I can't live without this!"

This is the Achilles' heel of any traditional quitting-cold-turkey plan, whether the substance of abuse is cocaine or gambling or a scoop of Cold Stone Creamery. And *this* is the critical moment that the Hunger Fix program helps you avoid. By keeping your body flush with dopamine during Detox, you'll never get a chance to feel that sense of stepping off the abstinence cliff. In the Hunger Fix plan, since you're not deprived of pleasure and reward, even if you do encounter that chocolate bar or bag of chips, your biologic reaction will not have that double rush of addictive delight. You're protected from the viselike grip of your False Fix, and you can quickly regroup. Your gradual rebuilding of dopamine receptors will be much more long lasting, much more sustainable, much more rewarding than simply detoxing cold turkey and leaving yourself wide open to withdrawal, then beating yourself up when you fall off the wagon.

Remember, you can never truly stay on the wagon in the traditional sense when your False Fix is food—you can't just stay away from the fridge the way you can a bar, casino, or crack house. That's why Stage 2 is all about keeping the dopamine boosted in the mesocortical dopamine system, the part of your brain that projects into the PFC, the zone more focused on, well, *focus.* Your working memory, motivation, organization, attention, and social behaviors all live here. In Stage 2, those new neurons will be constantly challenged to grow and increase the strength and complexity of your new Healthy Fix brain circuitry. Your buff new PFC then allows you to be able to sustain your Hunger Fix for life. Remember your mantra: Big Brain, Small Waist.

As you practice, practice, practice your basic Healthy Fix lifestyle habits, you'll strive for:

Progress, not perfection. Fight the addictive urge to aim for an all-or-nothing approach. Every single step, no matter the size, is a tremendous triumph.

Patience as you take it one day at a time to carefully integrate the mental, nutritional, and physical habits of your new Healthy Fix lifestyle.

Persistence as you hit life stresses that would normally drag you down into another False Fix binge. Embrace each slip as a golden opportunity to learn how to regroup without resorting to self-destruction and to continually refine your daily Healthy Fix habits.

Perseverance when the "inner addict" voices try to seduce you into believing their lies of immediate gratification. Quash them with your newly honed empowerment, reject the False Fixes, and choose your Healthy Hunger instead.

Presence, not mindlessness, in your own life. Paying attention, staying in the moment, and vigilance are essential to making the right decisions for self-care.

Power is your reward and your most potent weapon to control the cravings and addictive pushes and pulls that have kept you hostage for so long.

Practice now and for the rest of your life to strengthen and refine your Healthy Fixes, striving for mastery over your inner addict and its False Fixes. Through practice, you will find mastery.

Where You Are Now

In Stage 2, you'll continue to build upon the basic Healthy Fix blueprint you began to practice in Stage 1: Detox. You're now transitioning into beginner's recovery. What does that mean?

Your Clothes-O-Meter likely feels comfortable now, signaling that your body composition has improved. If you've not yet documented your body stats, now's the time. Turn to Appendix E and note your objective measures. If you took your baseline stats on day 1 of Detox, note your new numbers (record another self-video) and really let that sense of accomplishment sink in. See? You not only have more internal control over your False Fixes—your body composition has improved and it's time to choose the next size down.

From here, we're going to double down on your commitment to yourself. In Stage 2, your reward system has begun its recuperation process and your PFC is starting to strengthen to the point where you can set your sights a bit higher. If you have not already done so, I would like you to devise your Hunger Fix body quantity, quality, and size targets. (See the chart on page 317, Appendix E.) Once you've reached 80 percent of your Hunger Fix targets—and maintained them for 6 months—you'll move to Stage 3: Master Recovery. This is the stage of recovery you will remain in for the rest of your life.

This process might feel overwhelming, so remember: Recovery happens in *all* parts of our lives. We recover from financial distress, from divorces, from hurricane damage, from the death of a loved one. One of my friends calls herself a "recovering Catholic. Oh, the guilt I still drag around!" All of these experiences leave indelible memories, and each makes us stronger in its own way.

Life is all about recovery—wrap your food addiction right into the mix. Through a combination of family genetics passed on to you, and/or the epigenetic alterations caused by your earlier behavior, your biology and psychology are permanently changed. You hold an indelible memory for the taste of your False Fix, a memory only magnified if you have cross-addictions. So let's be frank: There is no cure. There is only a lifetime of freeing, rejuvenating, and joyful recovery.

One of my heroes is Betty Ford. I had the pleasure of working with her when I was the medical director of the Washington, DC, Race for the Cure for Breast Cancer. In addition to her assertive campaign to bring discussion of breast cancer into the public arena, she also courageously made public her battle with painkillers. Just listen to the Betty Ford Institute's definition of recovery: "Recovery is a voluntarily maintained lifestyle characterized by sobriety, personal health, and citizenship."

The Hunger Fix plan addresses recovery the same way: In Stage 1, you get "sober" from your False Fixes; in Stage 2, you build on this foundation of "personal health"; and, as you'll see later, Stage 3 moves you toward getting hooked on a helper's high, a richer engagement in your world, aka "citizenship."

Let's walk you through the portal of Stage 2 and learn more strategies to power up that PFC.

Update Your Hunger Fix Video Journal

Take a moment right now to update your Hunger Fix video journal. In your first video, you talked about your EpiphaME and your Healthy Hunger. Then you did your day 1 of Detox entry as well as regular check-ins, talking out loud about the challenges and triumphs along the way. Now it's time for another monologue as you transition to Stage 2. Ask yourself:

What are my feelings right now? Anticipation? Fear? Anxiety? Excitement?

What's my Healthy Hunger and what does it mean to me right now?

What are my expectations?

What is my vision of success?

What have I learned about myself?

What have I learned about my own False Fixes and addiction?

These clips are priceless motivators and humble reminders of where you came from and where you dream to go. If you're still camera shy, simply grab your written journal and let your words rip. Don't censor. Lay down your thoughts, feelings, and visions. Take another photo of yourself to go along with your notes. Make it a happy, positive, fun picture, filled with hope and self-appreciation. Share with me at www.drpeeke.com.

Stage 2: Mind

All habits involve brain adaptations—knee-jerk unconscious responses—that occur mindlessly. Through repetition, we have practiced certain actions and drilled them into our heads. Automatically wetting your toothbrush before (or after) you put on the toothpaste, or turning on the blinker before taking a turn, or checking your e-mail when you boot up your computer—these are your defaults. You don't have to think about them, you just do them—and it can feel very odd *not* to do them.

While most of our lives function on autopilot, the PFC is the part of our brain that helps guide us as we make choices—what to pay attention to, how to plan the day, how to make decisions and stay organized and intentional in our actions. Simply the act of *not* doing something you always do—and making another choice—can challenge and stretch your PFC, stimulating neural growth in this part of your brain.

In Stage 2, you'll learn to be proactive by creating and using alternate Healthy Fix coping strategies *before* stress hits. If we are vulnerable to stress, our False Fix is just waiting to draw us back to the candy aisle. That's why we have to short-circuit this whole cycle.

Keep chanting, "Victory through vigilance!" If you're in a stressful situation, at the first sign of your thinking that food will be the answer, you must continue to scream and shout, *"It's a lie!"*

Predictably, most people look for wiggle room with their False Fixes, and most likely you'll learn the hard way that there isn't any. That's okay—that lesson is part of the learning process. But pop right back up again, because vigilance is the key to long-term success—and there's solid science to prove this point.

The "successful losers" of the National Weight Control Registry (NWCR), a renowned ongoing study of people who have shed on average 66 pounds and kept the weight off on average for 5.5 years,

I Need a Fix

Watch Out for "Tim Tation"

Think of what powered you through Detox. There's usually a combination of mental pain and angst, anger and despair at hitting rock bottom, dogged determination, and hope. Once this amalgam reaches critical levels, nothing will get in your way. So here you are, using your new Healthy Fix habits to begin to shed excess body weight, and you're still feeling great. But watch out. As you enter Stage 2, some of that honeymoon glow of your starting weeks is going to fade. It has to. The novelty wears thin, and there you are, surrounded by all of your predictable False Fix triggers.

My patient Monique, a vivacious 50-year-old techie by day and spectacular soprano by night, put it this way:

> The eating IS getting better and I appreciate your e-mailed reminders! Bread and "no value" carbs are the enemy of Will Power (the guy I'm trying to let into my life). My old boyfriend, "Tim Tation," is so happy when my mind isn't engaged and fully participating (consciously) in my decision-making process. Rat bastard!! He won't leave me alone. I'm hoping Will Power will muscle up and help me kick Tim Tation out of my life (or at least out of my line o' sight, since we all know Tim Tation always hangs out looking to insinuate himself into any situation).

She should know. One year out from bariatric surgery (a sleeve gastrectomy), Monique is down 100 pounds of the 150 pounds she needs to shed. Monique realizes that while this surgery did save her life, GI surgery is not brain surgery—she knows that she, like anyone striving to shed unwanted body fat, had to engage her mind to combat her typical compulsive and addictive eating habits.

Typically, about 12 to 18 months after weight-loss surgery, many men and women notice that their appetite comes back and they are very susceptible to food cues, triggers, and temptation. Monique was no exception. Aware of her awakening appetite, she ramped up her efforts to plan her daily meals and snacks and not to default to old mindless grab-and-go habits. Her meditation and exercise are supporting her mental and physical strategy to rein in, and finally control, a lifelong pattern of addictive eating. And her reward? She continues to shed both the mental and the physical weight.

have been intensely studied by Drs. Jim Hill and Rena Wing in an effort to understand the secrets of these extraordinary folks who seem to have defied the odds. Their findings are perfectly in line with your Hunger Fix Recovery program:

- 94 percent of successful losers increased their physical activity, with the most frequently reported form of activity being walking.
- 78 percent eat breakfast every day.
- 75 percent weigh themselves and keep some kind of tracking at least once a week.
- 62 percent watch less than 10 hours of TV per week.
- 90 percent exercise, on average, about 1 hour per day, burning approximately 400 calories.

The successful losers have kept off from 30 to 300 pounds for anywhere from 1 to 66 years. Some lost the weight rapidly; others lost the weight very slowly (over as many as 14 years!). I had the opportunity to interview some of these men and women, and I was impressed with two general facts:

1. **Successful losers make serious changes to their living environments.** The majority of people in the NWCR made significant alterations to the persons, places, and things that did not support their new lifestyle habits. Every one of your daily, moment-to-moment choices and behaviors modify how your genes communicate with every cell in your body; all elements of your environment influence this conversation. Scrutinize how and where you live. Make strategic changes that support and maintain your Healthy Hunger rather than tempt you back into False Fixes.

2. **Successful losers are vigilant.** Some may even say hypervigilant. But I understand why they're so on top of their meals, weights, and exercise. Through the school of hard knocks, they have learned that if they let up enough and drop their vigilance, they'll succumb to temptation and significant weight regain. The longer they practice their new lifestyle, the more natural their daily vigilance

becomes. This orientation is no different from an alcoholic always scanning the environment, making certain he or she is "safe" from temptation. The longer the alcoholic is sober, the easier this becomes, but the vigilance can never, ever, under any circumstances, be completely dropped.

Learn how to self-mediate. Eating better and getting active are the low-hanging fruit of most weight-management programs. They're the elements most people are used to dealing with. However, we already know that "eat less, move more" is never, ever, going to be enough. Your mind is the master ruler.

How do I know this? Recall that in Chapter 5 I told you about my own journey and that I am now a consistent meditator, specifically using the simple Transcendental Meditation technique. The goal of TM is transcendence. This occurs when your mind settles inward beyond thought to experience the source of thoughts—pure awareness, also known as transcendental consciousness. This is the most silent and peaceful level of consciousness—your innermost self. In this state of restful alertness, your brain functions with significantly greater coherence and your body gains deep rest.

I was so intrigued by the newly emerging research showing the power of meditation to support addiction recovery, I decided to initiate a pilot study using TM in my patients with documented food addiction (all of whom completed the Yale Food Addiction Scale). In every case, the men and women who began to meditate noticed they were more calm as they confronted stress in their lives. Here's what Monique, my patient struggling to break up with "Tim Tation," said:

> The timing of integrating TM into my life couldn't be better. I tell you, the mental and physical challenges of the past few weeks have culminated in a big ol' pot of poo, and while it's stressful, I'm a lot calmer in response (already) and haven't immediately responded

with the automatic hand-to-mouth reflex that I've
refined over the past 40+ years.

My patients also stated that after 1 month, the meditation became
a daily oasis of peace and mental centering. Whenever they skipped
even a day, they were more aware of their addictive urges and had a
definite sense of loss of control over their False Fixes.

What's going on here?

Turns out that when people engage in regular meditation, they
release up to 65 percent more dopamine in the ventral striatum.[1] One
study found these increased levels of dopamine, and the continued
practice of mediation, reduced people's impulsiveness.[2] This alone
could help to put distance between you and the impulse to indulge in
your False Fixes. Remember the "three I's" (impulsivity, impatience,
and irritability)? Well, in addition to reining in your impulsive urges
to snag a False Fix and reawaken your addiction, meditation will also
ramp up your patience and smooth out your mood.

People with addictive tendencies spend so much time either desperately seeking their False Fix or laid out in a False Fix coma, they have
no enjoyment of the amazing things going on around them. Meditation increases the pleasure and reward of the sensory experiences
from Healthy Fixes—aka "living in the moment." Savoring the sensual delight of a smoothie or a veggie-and-cheese-filled omelet, or
hiking to the top of a mountain: Each of these pleasurable adventures
is experienced more deeply with meditation-driven mindfulness.

Meditation also helps prevent relapse. An fMRI study done at the
University of California in San Francisco found that people who were
least likely to relapse in alcoholic abstinence programs were those with
greater brain volume and thicker cortices throughout the reward system. They had a much easier time sticking with their sobriety—and
when they fell off the wagon, they experienced less severe relapse.[3]
And, as you learned in Detox, meditation stimulates neurogenesis,

especially in the PFC. More than 600 medical studies have found that Transcendental Meditation is scientifically proven to:

- Improve memory, problem solving, and functioning in the brain's left hemisphere (verbal and analytic thinking) and right hemisphere (synthetic and holistic thinking).

- Increase blood flow to the brain, flexibility of brain functioning, and efficiency of information transfer to the brain.

- Mobilize latent reserves of the brain and speed up reaction times.

- Increase intelligence in secondary and college students and improve academic performance.

- Accelerate cognitive development in children.

- Increase creativity, self-confidence, tolerance, and efficiency of perception.

- Increase muscle relaxation and improve response to stress.

- Increase resistance to distraction and social pressure.

- Improve relationships.

- Decrease hostility, cortisol, cholesterol, blood pressure, insulin resistance, insomnia, anxiety, and depression.

- Decrease medical costs.

Comedian Russell Brand credits TM with helping him break his addictions to heroin, sex, and alcohol.[4] And celebrities from Brand to Ellen DeGeneres to Jerry Seinfeld have all teamed up with the David Lynch Foundation to spread the word about the benefits of TM. Speaking to the *New York Times*, filmmaker Lynch said meditation can give us everything that's "missing from life today: unbounded intelligence, creativity, bliss, love, energy, peace. Things like tension, anxieties, traumatic stress, sorrow, depression, hate, rage, need for revenge, fear—poooft!—all this starts to lift away."[5]

Or try mindfulness-based stress reduction. There are so many meditation options available to you, from the relaxation response to mind centering to monastic, from Zen to breath conscious. I encourage you to do what I did—check a few of them out and experiment to see what might fit you the best. (See Appendix F for a full list of meditation options and contact information.)

Let's look at mindfulness-based stress reduction (or MBSR, or simply "mindfulness meditation"), another form of meditation practice that's been widely studied and found to have some of the same health benefits as TM. Made popular by Jon Kabat-Zinn, PhD, and other stress researchers, MBSR shares with TM the common mission to be present in the moment, creating space and time to look clearly at the persons, places, and things in one's life and their influence on the ability to make the right decision. Whereas TM's main goal is transcendence, MBSR's is to prioritize mindfulness in everyday life.

One study found that after an 8-week program, previous MBSR novices showed significant gains in the size of their brains, with the most gray matter growing in the posterior cingulate cortex, the temporo-parietal junction, and the cerebellum, brain regions that help us learn and remember, stay calm and not overreact emotionally, critically evaluate our own thoughts, and understand other people's perspectives.[6] Any method you use to generate neurogenesis helps you to stay clean and reduces the chance you will fall prey to other False Fixes— and growing these specific brain regions can help that much more.[7]

Mindfulness is simply the act of paying attention to the present moment, observing your thoughts and feelings, acknowledging them, and letting them go. You can do mindfulness meditation, but you can also do mindful walking, mindful swimming, even mindful eating! (You'll learn a mindfulness eating practice in the Stage 2: Mouth section.) To perform a mindfulness meditation, simply:

- Sit comfortably in a chair, or on the floor or a bed, with your legs crossed.
- Close your eyes.
- Breathe in through your nose and "observe" your breath, in and out.

the 20 words into the correct categories, then choose the original words out of a list of 180.

Can you believe simply doing these four exercises could improve your ability to withstand cravings, avoid your False Fixes, and focus more on your long-term goals? Amazing!

You can find hundreds of online or offline memory games (start with www.memorise.org/memory-gym, www.easysurf.cc/menu.htm, or www.lumosity.com) to increase your working memory—and there are other options as well. A study done in Japan found that people who spent time writing about traumatic events in their lives had improvements on tests of working memory.[13] And score another one for meditation: One study found improvements in working memory after just four meditation training sessions.[14]

Mind your macrocosm. In Detox, you began to take inventory of the persons, places, and things in your environment that either hinder or help your Hunger Fix lifestyle. You'll continue this process for the rest of your life, constantly scanning your living and working environments and staying vigilant about any cues, new or old, that may trigger your False Fixes. Whether it's scoping out where you'll go to lunch with a friend, a party, the office fridge, airplane food, or vacation celebrations, be on the lookout for unsafe surroundings. Cuing in your A^2 skills, adapt and adjust accordingly. You're in control. Even slight modifications can make a world of difference.

Establish your Stage 2 body weight-loss goal. You need to achieve 80 percent of your body weight-loss target and maintain it for 6 months before you can transition to Stage 3. During the 6 months, you can continue to shed more pounds. You may even fluctuate up and down by 5 to 10 pounds, because it's normal to bounce up and down a bit. But by the end of the 6 months, in order to consider yourself a master and move to Stage 3, you need to achieve at least 80 percent of your weight-loss goal.

Example: How to Transition through the Three Stages

Gender	Female
Height	5'4"
Starting Weight	200 lb
Starting Body Fat Percentage	39%
Hunger Fix Weight Goal	Remove 50 lb
Stage 1 Detox	
Detox Time Period	4 weeks
Body Weight Change	Removed 8 lb
Clothes-o-Meter	Down 1 size
Stage 2 Beginner Recovery	
Stage 2 Time Period	6½ months
Initial Stage 2 Body Weight Change	Removed 34 lb
Stage 2 Body Weight Change	42 lb (84% of goal)
Weight Change during 6-Month Waiting Period	Gained 5 lb, removed 10 lb
Stage 1 + 2 Net Combined Weight Removal	47 lbs (94% of goal)
Clothes-o-Meter	Down 5 dress sizes
Stage 3 Master Recovery	

How long will this take you to achieve? As with Detox, the time is variable. It depends on how much weight you have to remove as well as how many confounding personal and environmental variables you face in your unique journey. As much as you want to speed through this whole process, you can't. Please remember that the brain needs time to grow fresh new neurons; the goal is to remove weight and keep it off *for the rest of your life.*

Weight loss and maintenance are two distinctly different processes. Most folks will tell you that it's much easier to drop the weight than to maintain the loss. I have a golden rule: *The manner in which you dropped the weight in the first place will determine whether or not you'll be able to keep it off long-term.* That's why you need to approach your Healthy Fix lifestyle in a well-planned, gradual, and methodical manner. By doing so, you'll reap marvelous rewards along the way, and you'll know in your heart that you're building a powerful mental and physical foundation that will allow you to maintain your wonderful new weight for life.

Stage 2: Mouth

By following the Hunger Fix eating plan during Stage 1: Detox, you increased the amount of dopamine-boosting foods in your diet. Now we're going to expand your nutritional focus to support greater neurogenesis in the PFC. You'll also incorporate mindful eating exercises that will extend the neural benefits of your meditation practice (you'll make the Mind-Mouth connection) and help you key into the sensual pleasures of every bite you put in your mouth.

Important note: Even though you're feeling stronger now, the key is *not* to expose yourself to the foods you abuse again, or you awaken the False Fix demons once more. Stay as *far away* from your trigger cues as possible while you allow your brain to rebuild itself. As you get smarter and stronger, and as Stage 2 continues, your safe "smart relapses" become safer and smarter. When the going gets funky, you have an extra yogurt with berries and walnuts—or two. So what? It's *nothing* compared with what you used to do. The rule is that what you choose to do cannot lead to a feeling of being out of control followed by an all-out binge. It has to be a safe food you know will be a treat and added calories, perhaps driven by stress, but you'll be able to regroup and move on.

Let's look at some other ways to expand your Hunger Fix Mouth plan.

Reconnect with food through mindful eating. People who have gained weight over a 6-month period[15] or who carry the DRD2 A1 genetic allele experience a greater flood of dopamine in the gustatory cortex in response to the anticipation of eating delicious foods. But recall the tragic irony of repeated dopamine flooding: In spite of these high dopamine levels, these folks actually derive less pleasure as they eat, with less activity in the brain's dorsal striatum—causing them to eat more because they're looking for that high.[16] In other words, you want it more but end up enjoying it less, so you eat more to compensate, to try to get that "high" you once got from the same foods. Then that extra eating itself causes a decrease in your dopamine receptors—and the downward spiral continues.

But if you can slow down and really taste your food, experience each bite, you'll derive more pleasure out of the experience of eating. You'll quickly find you're satisfied with less. It takes time for the brain to process fullness signals, so slower eating allows for fullness to register in the brain so it can send out the "stop eating" message before you overeat. But people packing extra pounds tend to eat faster than slimmer folks—especially guys—and research suggests refined grains are consumed faster than whole grains. (They go down too easy!)

Not only is it easy to wolf down our meals when we're distracted by worries, urgency, or whatever's on TV at the moment, but the food industry actively encourages this tendency, says former FDA commissioner David Kessler, MD. In his book *The End of Overeating*, Dr. Kessler explains that food marketers design processed foods to be easy to chew and swallow, so we'll gulp them down before our appetite is sated, leading us to buy and consume more food than we need. That ease of eating is what makes some False Fix foods so insidious.

Mindful eating of natural whole foods helps counter this habit of wolfing down your food and, as a form of meditation, it can generate new brain cells and further plump up the cerebral cortex. Experiment with one Healthy Fix food at a time. Smell it, stare at it for a few moments—notice the colors, the presentation, the steam rising off the plate. Take a bite into your mouth, close your eyes, and really experience the flavors and the textures. This concentrated attention not only helps your body register fullness faster but may also help you rebuild your natural appreciation for and love of Healthy Fix foods.

Visualize your new Hunger Fix eating plan. When 177 students at McGill University set a goal to eat fruit over the course of the next 7 days, the students who visualized how, when, and where they would buy, prepare, and eat the fruit ended up eating twice as much fruit as those who just intended to do so. The lead researcher attributes the success of the visualization to the same types of mental rehearsal you see in sports psychology.[17]

Every morning before you get out of bed, take 5 minutes to watch yourself going through each meal and snack of the day. Where will you get it? How will you prepare it? Where will you eat it? Use this technique with other Healthy Fixes, like exercise. When will you walk the dog? How will you get the dog's leash? Where are your socks and sneakers? All of this information will make it that much more automatic for you to make the right choices during the day.

Create shopping, eating, and cooking rituals. So many addicts have food terrors—they're terrified of being near food and especially cooking because they're afraid they'll lose control. My aim is that you fall in love with food again, but in a healthy way, through simple cooking, or reconnecting with cooking at a very simple level.

Establishing rituals to support healthy eating is essential. Lack of organization will feed into the chaotic, addictive False Fix lifestyle pattern. Rituals provide structure. The trick is to ritualize your eating as much as possible—when you shop for food, how you prepare your meals, and the how-when-where you eat your meals and snacks.

You can transform any Healthy Fix into a ritual that can neutralize a False Fix. For example, to neutralize late-night eating, create an herbal-tea-making ritual at 7:45 p.m. to signal to your mind that you choose not to eat past 8:00. As you take your tea into a comfortable room, turn off the lights in the kitchen, "shutting it down" for the evening.

Stay out of the kitchen! You heard me. When you're not preparing foods for your meals or snacks, steer clear of the kitchen. Even kitchens that are pristine and cleansed of all False Fixes still harbor permanent cues and triggers for most people. The kitchen can be a safe haven when you're there for a Healthy Fix purpose. Otherwise, you'll find yourself picking and grazing and potentially triggering a relapse.

Here's a novel approach one of my patients shared with me. A 45-year-old busy working mom, Helen grew up in a household with five siblings. Her mom grew tired of cleaning up the mess left when kids kept streaking through her kitchen. So her dad carved a wooden sign that read KITCHEN CLOSED on one side and KITCHEN OPEN on the other. Once any meal or snack ritual was over, the closed sign appeared and there was hell to pay if you were caught sneaking in for a treat, especially at nighttime. Lo and behold, as an adult, this early mental conditioning resulted in Helen's never having problems with extracurricular adventures to the kitchen, especially postdinner. Her "normal" was to avoid the kitchen then. Instead, her challenge was overeating in the midafternoon when she returned from work and was preparing snacks for the kids. She learned to become more vigilant during her trigger hours in the afternoon, to plan a healthy midafternoon snack, to avoid any False Fix foods, and to stop eating her kids' snacks. (Oh, and by the way, she created her own kitchen sign to pass on this valuable ritual to her children.)

Establish new ways to work around food. And as you've seen, the new rules apply as much to *when* you're actually in the kitchen as well as what you're doing while you prepare your meals.

Chew your food! This may sound like unnecessary advice; of course you chew your food! But try paying attention the next time you're eating; you may be surprised to find that you're not doing as much chewing as you think you are. Especially if you're in a rush, as we all too often are when we eat. A small study done in China reveals a tangible benefit that springs from making this simple change to your eating habits. When scientists tested 30 volunteers, they found that the obese subjects chewed less and ate faster. However, when the researchers had their subjects chew their food 40 times, allowing them to eat as much or little as they wished, the diners ended up ingesting 11 percent fewer calories. This was true for both obese and lean test subjects. Imagine, cutting your calorie intake by over 10 percent, just by chewing more! In the study, blood tests revealed that more chewing was associated with lower levels of ghrelin, a hormone that increases appetite and may affect dopamine-sensitive cells in the brain.[18]

Expand your diet to include more PFC-building foods. You've now spent considerable time keeping dopamine levels high with Stage 1 foods, especially because of the emphasis on amino acids tyrosine and phenylalanine. Indeed, a double-blind placebo-controlled study at the University of Cambridge School of Medicine found that supplementation with tyrosine and phenylalanine helped depressed people improve their mood, speed of thought, and interest in completing tasks. Researchers attributed these improvements directly to the effect the tyrosine and phenylalanine had on their dopamine levels. Interestingly, though, the subjects' frontal cortex function was unchanged.

That's not to say that your PFC has not benefited from all the amazing nutrients you've been downing—but in Stage 2, you're going to broaden your food palette to bring in more varied "brain food," foods that will provide your brain with the raw materials for robust neurogenesis in the PFC. Especially important are foods that naturally increase serotonin, the calming neurotransmitter that helps your emotions stay on an even keel so you can make wise, forward-thinking Stage 2 decisions.

Choline[19] is the precursor to the acetylcholine, another neurotransmitter in the nucleus accumbens (NA) that plays a part in our feeling sated after a meal. Medications that control appetite release acetylcholine in the NA, and researchers believe these medications may also help people who abuse drugs such as cocaine and heroin. Even your body's own appetite suppressants, the calming neurotransmitter serotonin and peptide hormone cholecystokinin (CCK), get much of their hunger-fighting power from aceytylcholine.[20]

Choline also figures prominently in attention and the prefrontal cortex. Studies on rats have shown that supplementing with dietary choline can increase the nerve growth factor in the prefrontal cortex,[21] improving their memory and precision, helping reduce aging deficits[22] and even bouncing back from early PFC injury.[23] Acetylcholine is also credited with strengthening synapses, the connections between neurons, particularly when you're learning and using your short-term memory.[24]

We make a small amount of choline in our bodies, but we would be deficient if we didn't get more from food. Choline also helps protect against liver cancer, memory loss, and Alzheimer's.

Foods High in Choline

Meat and Eggs	Top round, chuck roast, bottom round, beef brisket, top sirloin, tenderloin, eggs (especially egg yolks)
Dairy	Butter, milk
Vegetables	Potatoes, cauliflower, tomatoes
Fruits	Banana, oranges
Nuts and Seeds	Sesame seeds, flaxseeds
Legumes and Beans	Soy lecithin, soybeans and soybean products, peanuts and peanut butters, lentils
Whole Grains	Oats, barley, corn, whole wheat bread
Extras	Ginseng root

Omega-3s are used by the brain to form 60 percent of its fat-based cell structure. These fatty acids ensure that cell membranes will be flexible enough to allow other nutrients in. One study found that rats fed a diet low in omega-3s had 20 percent lower levels of the omega-3 docosahexaenoic acid (DHA), which researchers found significantly reduced the density of the D2 dopamine receptors in the ventral striatal section of the brain—an area closely associated with impulsivity. Another study found that supplementing with fish oil increased the activation of serotonin receptors and increased the production of BDNF in the hippocampus, actions that scientists believe help improve memory and decrease anxiety and depression.

Perhaps the best way to test how omega-3s can influence our ability to calm down and focus is to go to the zaniest, most scattered source: 8- to 10-year-old boys. One placebo-controlled fMRI study found that supplementing with DHA for 8 weeks increased activity in the boys' dorsolateral prefrontal cortex significantly more than placebo. The study also found a "dose response"—the more DHA the boys had taken, the higher the concentration in their brain, the greater the activity in their PFC, and the faster their reaction times had become.[25] Not bad for a little fish oil, huh?

Foods High in Omega-3s

Meat and Eggs	Caviar, sardines, mackerel, salmon, whitefish, anchovies, herring, oysters, halibut, scallops, shrimp, tuna, cod, striped bass, rainbow trout, snapper, organic free-range beef, omega-3 enriched eggs
Dairy	Omega-3 enriched milk
Vegetables	Romaine lettuce, spinach, collard greens, kale, summer squash, turnip greens, winter squash, brussels sprouts, green beans, canned grape leaves, cauliflower, arugula
Fruits	Raspberries, strawberries
Nuts and Seeds	Flaxseed oil, flaxseeds, chia seeds, radish seeds, butternuts, walnuts, walnut oil, mustard seeds, alfalfa seeds
Legumes and Beans	Edamame, tofu, miso, soybean mayonnaise
Whole Grains	Uncle Sam cereal, wheat germ oil
Extras	Fish oil capsules, basil, oregano, cloves, marjoram, tarragon, spearmint, canned capers, yellow mustard, Caesar dressing

Expand your diet to include other "brain foods." Widen your view to other foods that support and feed your PFC—and there are many! The beautiful part of this plan is that it's all you need to have a nutritionally optimal diet for life. Every single food that's good for your brain is good for your entire body.

- **Beta-carotene** counters the oxidative stress that can age the brain prematurely. *Good sources include* sweet potatoes, carrots, kale, spinach, turnip greens, winter squash, collard greens.

- **Vitamin B$_{12}$** and other B vitamins play an essential role by allowing nerve cells to develop properly and by helping to manufacture and release neurotransmitters. *Good sources include* yellowfin tuna, chicken breast, sardines, snapper, salmon, beef tenderloin, lamb, scallops, shrimp, halibut, bell peppers, turnip greens, spinach.

- **Vitamin C** is an antioxidant that helps protect brain cells from free-radical damage brought on by toxins in our environment. *Good sources include* strawberries, papaya, bell peppers, broccoli, brussels sprouts, oranges, cantaloupe, kiwifruit, cauliflower, kale.

- **Zinc** helps balance blood sugar and plays a critical role as a catalyst for neurotransmitter creation. *Good sources include* beef tenderloin, lamb loin, chickpeas, sesame seeds, pumpkin seeds, low-fat yogurt, turkey, peas.

Stage 2: Muscle

Transitioning through Detox, you experienced your body's own unique response to movement. For some of you, it has been an athletic reawakening, and your brain is kicking back into gear as you recall how good your body used to feel. For others, physical activity has never been an important piece of life, and therefore it's a novel experience. Regardless of your background, the key lesson throughout the Healthy Fix lifestyle is that you will never, ever control the overeating and food addiction struggle, nor will you achieve your healthiest dream weight and maintain it for life, *unless you incorporate physical activity in your life*. Recall the data from the National Weight Control Registry. Those "successful losers" burned on average 400 calories per day, and the mainstay of their activity is walking, not an Olympic boot camp.

Also, notice that I don't love to use the word *exercise*. I just want you to get up and move. Do whatever you like, but get vertical, get going, and keep it going for life! Activities of daily living—cleaning up, washing the car—count big-time, so never discount them. For those of you who don't break out into hives when the "E" word is mentioned, rock on with whatever you love to do, whether it's joining a softball team, a spin class, or a heart-thumping wild and crazy Zumba class.

You may have been tentative about physical activity in Detox, but in Stage 2 it's gonna become a part of your life. *With every step and every drop of sweat, you're building a more powerful brain as you're pushing yourself further and further away from your False Fixes.* Getting physical is not an option anymore. It must become a nonnegotiable part of your life. Remember the mantra: Big Brain, Small Waist.

John Ratey, MD, from Harvard calls exercise "Miracle-Gro for the brain." Exercise or physical activity of all kinds—cardio, strength training, yoga, dancing—stimulates neurogenesis, partly thanks to that amazing brain-derived neurotrophic factor (BDNF). One study published in the journal *Neuroscience* found that just 1 week of rat cardio—on the wheel—resulted in a 171 percent increase in the amount of BDNF in the rodents' brains. The BDNF was also proved to grow more neurons in the hippocampus—the intensity of the exercise was directly related to the number of neurons that are activated in the dentate gyrus of the hippocampus.[26] Once rats have become accustomed to regular exercise, if they're prevented from doing it, they'll experience a craving that shows up in the reward system, the same way that a chocoholic's brain would crave a Dove bar.

In Stage 2, you'll experiment and try out new experiences—Zumba class, Spinning, couch–to–5-K programs—that challenge your muscles while their novelty or competitive zing triggers extra dopamine release. Mainly, like the other M's, Stage 2: Muscle is all about practice, practice, practice. Having established the regular habit of exercise in Stage 1, now you're trying to increase duration so you can build stamina and willpower. Whatever you have to do to make sure that habit sticks, do it!

Know your five active body rewards. As your mind and body continue to withdraw from False Fixes and latch onto Healthy Fixes like physical activity, you'll learn more about the importance of your five active body rewards: endurance (cardio), strength (weight lifting), core (strong torso and abs), flexibility (stretching), and balance.

As you leave your old mind-body dissociation behind and move toward forming a powerfully positive mental and physical cycle, you need to stay physically active. In Stage 1: Detox, I asked you to take it easy and gradually increase your activity. This made you feel better, and gave you more energy. Now you're going to take it up a notch and discover more endurance through cardio activities and strength training. Both require you to engage your core, do some stretching, and count on your balance. You're hitting all five active body rewards. We'll take them a step further in Stage 3.

Frequency. In the best of worlds, you want to stay active every day of your life. But you often don't live in the best of worlds. So you'll want to aim for at least 5 days a week when you can schedule 20 to 30 minutes of increasingly intense activity. Meanwhile, all day long, in addition to your scheduled activity time, find every opportunity you can to assume the vertical. Why? To avoid what James Levine, MD, at the Mayo Clinic has coined "sitting disease." People who sit glued to any tube or screen for more than 4 hours per day have a significantly increased risk of diabetes, heart disease, and cancer.[27] So get up, people!

- **Fidget.** When you're sitting and cannot get up, fidget as much as you can. It burns calories and keeps your muscles moving.

- **Torque it.** If your back can handle it, sit on an ab or stability ball instead of a desk chair. You'll constantly extend and contract multiple muscles as well as engage your core.

- **Walkin 'n' talkin.** Stuck talking on the phone all day? Grab a headset and move around while you talk. Instead of sitting through a client meeting, suggest taking a walk. Or if a friend wants to talk, suggest a walk. Before you know it, you'll be racking up the calorie burn, shedding fat, and beefing up your PFC—and probably enjoying your conversations a lot more!

- **Ditch the guilt.** Women in particular feel it's not right to take time out for self-care, and if they do, they quickly erase it from their calendar with the first cry for help from a friend, family member, neighbor, whomever. If you want to achieve the mind and body you deserve and manage your addiction for life, you have got to flip this guilt on its head. Protect your active time with all of your might. Schedule it and make it a priority. For those who feel guilty if they're away from their desk or family for too long, try what one of my patients did. She simply made up a "Susan" in the next building and needed to get up out of her seat, take the stairs, and leave her building to see this person frequently for her work. No one cared, and she never made a big deal about it. Six months later and 25 pounds lighter, she's the one laughing all the way to the size 10 aisle.

HIIT IT. Even just a quick few minutes of dancing can snap yourself out of a craving. If you dance with intensity and you sweat, you trigger the same reward pathways as addictive drugs, increasing the concentration of dopamine in your brain.[28] In fact, a study from Wake Forest University found that really cutting loose and dancing your butt off will give you all the cardiovascular benefits that a treadmill running session will.[29]

By increasing the sweat or intensity of your physical activity, you'll spend less time and get more out of it. This is all relative to your starting place right now. Two or three times a week, increase the intensity of your cardio and do it in intervals. This is called high intensity interval training (HIIT). So if you've been sedentary, simply warm up for 5 to 10 minutes, then increase your speed and/or hill incline so you're working harder. Do this for 1 to 3 minutes, then come back to a moderate pace for 2 minutes, then increase to the higher intensity level. Keep that pace rotation up for 20 to 30 minutes and you'll have accomplished more than if you'd trudged like a zombie for an hour. One small study of people with type 2 diabetes found that exercising very intensely for just 10 minutes within a 25-minute cardio workout three times a week lowered participants' blood sugar and reduced their postmeal blood glucose spikes. This program also boosted their muscles' mitochondrial proteins, a source of power for cells that helps improve your body composition.[30] Bumping up your intensity saves time, gives you much more energy for your time and sweat, and helps grow those precious PFC neurons.

Fit it in. To get the most of out of walking, or any cardio, you need to:

- **Schedule it:** Whip out a pen or your smartphone and write down what time you'll get out and hoof it, whether it's in the neighborhood or at the gym. Writing it down says you mean it and ascribes respect and honor to this task.

- **Make it a reward:** There will always be constant interruptions and distractions to drag you away from your appointed time. Flip your feelings about getting physical on their head. Look at it as a gift to yourself, some sacred time when no one can bother you. This will help you reclaim your hijacked reward system.

- **Get creative:** One of my patients works at the Pentagon, which is 1 mile around. A busy mom and full-time assistant to a general, she simply donned walking shoes and instead of shooting e-mails to the folks on the other side of the Pentagon, she walked to them whenever she could. One year and 30 fewer pounds later, she was down four dress sizes, feeling fit and energized, and her behavior went viral. Now a group of her co-workers are literally following in her footsteps. Looking in the mirror, she sees the reward. The junk she used to eat and her past sedentary lifestyle suddenly don't feel so rewarding anymore.

Track it. If you want a sense of accomplishment, especially if you're a beginning exerciser, then log your laps. Scope out your progress every week and give yourself a pat on the back. There are many cool apps out there to track your physical activity as well as help motivate you. See Appendix F.

Put some muscle into it. If you're gung-ho on cardio, why do you need to strengthen your body as well? The reason is that you're doing two different things. Cardio helps keep your heart—a four-chambered muscle—in excellent healthy shape while also burning excess fat. Strength training keeps your calorie-burning engine red hot so that for every step you take while you're walking, you're optimizing the number of calories you cook. It's like going from a puny 4-cylinder engine to a burning-hot 8-cylinder Formula 1 racing car. Rev it up!

Strength training also puts some muscle mass on your PFC: In a 12-month randomized controlled trial of older women who did resistance training just once or twice a week, their selective attention and ability to handle conflict—executive functions handled by the PFC—increased by almost 13 percent.[31] Plus, your body will never ever look tight, compact, lean, and muscular unless you add strength training. The great news is that you can do it at home, on the road, or in a health club. Most of the time you just need your body to make it work. If you're new to strength training, here are a few tips:

- **Find a fitness professional to show you the basics.** This can be done cheaply if you join a group at the community center or take a class that emphasizes weight training (check out www.ideafit.com/fitnessconnect). Or rustle up a friend or two and pay for a trainer to show you correct form. Another option is to purchase one of the many great DVDs and apps out there with specific instruction for beginners as well as more advanced folks. Achieving and maintaining good form is imperative and will help you reduce the risk of injury.

- **Make it a home experience.** In my books *Fit to Live* and *Body for Life for Women,* I presented simple at-home exercises you can do to lay down an effective foundation for strengthening your muscles. Simply purchase a full-length mirror that you can lean against the wall, a floor mat, some elastic tubing with handles, a chair, and hand weights and you're in business. (See Appendix F for other resources.)

- **Don't worry about bulking up!** First, let me tell you that you're not going to become a bodybuilder overnight. This is one of the most common misconceptions about strength training. You will simply become more lean and toned. Second, please be patient and perseverant as you enjoy your regular weight-lifting sessions. Age, gender, past body composition, and past athletic history all factor into this equation. It takes time to change your body composition. Those with patience will indeed be rewarded with stronger willpower as well: One study found just a 12-week resistance-training regimen made smokers twice as likely to be able to quit compared with those who didn't lift weights.[32]

- **Twice or thrice a week does it.** Plan on doing some form of strength training for about 30 minutes, two or three times per week. Try not to train on consecutive days, as your body needs time to adapt and adjust in the interim. Leaving 2 days in between is optimal for beginners. And as you improve, keep challenging yourself: One study found that the greater your muscle mass, the healthier your body's response to insulin and the lower your risk of developing type 2 diabetes.[33]

Stick to simple. Many of my most successful patients have found ways to move their bodies and have stuck to a basic, easy-to-follow recipe. Whether it's getting that walk in every day, or playing tennis three times a week with a buddy, or swimming early in the morning at the indoor county pool, or just hopping on an elliptical, they've all found a tolerable and even enjoyable way to get their physical activity done. Many don't veer too far away and experiment because they figure if they got great results from doing their program, why mess with it? Hey, whatever works for you is fine with me.

Push It Up

One exercise that you need to know, and my personal secret: the push-up. Traditional name: close grip push-up. I love push-ups because you can hit six muscles at once—shoulder, chest, biceps, triceps, abs, and glutes. Even the back gets engaged. What's not to love? Get into a push-up position on the floor and place your hands directly under your shoulders. It's perfectly fine to do a bent-knee push-up if you cannot do this exercise with a straight leg. For that matter, if you have problems with your elbows, just do the exercise off the wall by stepping back a pace or two and leaning into the wall.

Keeping elbows in by your side, and with your face up and looking forward, lower your body down for a count of two. Then straighten your arms and return to start. Don't forget to engage your core by contracting your ab muscles and squeezing your butt as you do each push-up. Even if you can do only one or two with great form, that's a terrific start in Stage 2. See if you can slowly but surely work your way to 10.

Learn a new discipline. There are folks who love to play around and find new ways to cross-train. This means you continue to do your baseline rhythmic cardio, your walking/elliptical/running or whatever, but you now add a new experience—Pilates, yoga, martial arts, cycling, Spinning, rowing, swimming, weight training, Zumba, hip-hop, jump rope, belly dancing—anything that stimulates new mental learning, and thus neurogenesis, while actually physically moving (yet more neurogenesis!). We're looking to have fun, for crying out loud. With fun comes pleasure and a tsunami of dopamine. Spice it up! Variety will continue to delight your dopamine center— the surprise of the new will get your synapses firing and will gratify that need for a "rush."

Club it up. Want to meet Healthy Hunger tribal members? There are so many options for health clubs, including 24/7 health clubs open at all hours to meet your unique schedule needs. Morning larks and night owls unite! One of my favorite clubs is Anytime Fitness, whose founder, Chuck Runyon, wrote a terrific book, *Working Out Sucks!* The book is highly motivating for folks who consider physical activity some kind of boot camp nightmare. And if you love the motto "no men, no makeup, no mirrors," there's Curves, with their new Curves Complete lifestyle program and strong emphasis on dropping inches with weight training and cardio. Meet up with other like-minded ladies and let it rip. They even have Zumba classes now. And don't forget to check out YMCA/YWCA clubs across the country, along with your local neighborhood community centers. Log onto www.active.com and scope out countless recreational and sports activities in every community. There are endless Healthy Fix resources in the health club world.

Watch the news while working out. Do those talking heads segments on news channels stir you up and make you angry or frustrated? Watching something that incites your ire can increase levels of dopamine. A study published in the journal *Neuroreport* found that when subjects were hooked up to PET machines and shown inflammatory words, the emotional response resulted in an increase of dopamine compared to neutral words. The authors speculate that dopamine helps us assign a value to the objects that trigger our emotions in our memories—thus enabling our brains to learn from these anger-inducing experiences.[34] No wonder people like to fight about politics! Channel this energy into your next workout on the treadmill, stationary bike, or elliptical machine.

Explore your outside world. You were encouraged to hug a tree or two during Detox. Let's keep the momentum going. Start with your walks, but move on to hikes in lovely surroundings you can walk or drive to. Researchers in at the University of Michigan found that people who went for a walk in a natural setting, or even viewed pictures of nature, performed better on memory tests (but people who walked on a busy street did not). Our brains seem to delight in the sights and sounds of nature. The Japanese have a name for this outdoor immersion: *shinrin-yoku*, or "forest bathing." A study of people at 24 Japanese forests found that just 15-minute walks in the forest lowered concentrations of cortisol, pulse rate, blood pressure and enhanced parasympathetic and sympathetic nervous system function.[35] Indeed, a Korean fMRI study found that simply *looking* different images of nature and city life provoked different reactions in our brains. Cityscapes activated the amygdala, the seat of instinctive base reactions such as fear, a reaction that indicated anxiety. But images of green spaces activated the anterior cingulated gyrus, the site of anticipation and empathy, and the caudate nucleus, a part of the brain saturated with dopamine neurons.

If you don't have a forest or nature preserve nearby, go local. Spend your lunch break exploring the neighborhood around your office. Find a walking path and do loops for 30 minutes, or do lunges across your backyard. Even reading a book outside in a green space will help you focus and regulate yourself (but don't forget to get up and move around between chapters!). One study found that inner-city girls who had a view of a green space from their windows at home had greater self-discipline than those who did not. And the greener her view, the more a girl could concentrate, the longer she could resist temptations and delay gratification, and the lower her levels of impulsivity—all actions controlled by the PFC.[36] Anything to get outside!

Shed some light on yourself. You may have heard of people using light therapy—exposure to bright light—to counteract seasonal depression. There's evidence that bright light stimulates production of the neurochemical serotonin, a key neurotransmitter for proper functioning of the PFC and general brain functioning. Studies have found that people have higher serotonin levels during summer than in winter, and one study found that women low on tryptophan maintained a positive mood if they were exposed to bright light during the day. The take-home message: Our brains work best when our bodies get plenty of sunlight. And it's not just a seasonal thing; we spend so much time indoors that for many of us, the sun exposure we get during the summer is less than what our ancestors used to get during the short days of winter.

If you're sun starved, you could try using specialized lights intended to treat seasonal depression to help your PFC generate the serotonin it needs.[37] Those lamps can be expensive or impractical, though (some generate 60 times as much illumination as typical home lighting does). The Center for Environmental Therapeutics offers a tabletop model at www.cet.org.[38] An easier solution: Make sure to spend some time outside every day, as often as you can, all year round. Take the long way when you walk the dog; pass some time with a neighbor across the fence; institute a daily family stroll around the neighborhood; eat lunch on a park bench or at an outdoor café. Sunlight not only keeps your brain humming with serotonin but also helps your body produce vitamin D, a nutrient many of us are lacking. And if you spend some of your outdoor time in a natural setting, even a park

Do a "Perfect" Day

Here's a little experiment for you: Today, try to do everything absolutely *perfectly*. From the moment you wake up until the moment you go to bed, do your absolute best not to mess up even once. Count every calorie; exercise exactly as much as you had planned, to the minute. I'll bet you that most people can't last very long. Worse, they end up berating themselves for not achieving "perfection." That perfectionism and inflexibility are exactly why 95 percent of us struggle to keep the weight off.

Just remember that *perfectionism equals paralysis*. You can't move forward when you're afraid to make a single mistake. Bag any pursuit of perfection and instead opt for progress instead. Be kind to yourself and allow flexibility for your own humanity. You've run the "perfect" experiment. Now swear off perfectionism right now, okay?

---

or backyard, you'll get the stress-busting benefits of being in nature.

Play Wii Fit. A British study published in the journal *Nature* found that increases in dopamine during video game playing are equivalent to the boost that would occur if you were to shoot up with amphetamines.[39] To get the natural high, try a vigorous game of Wii Fit to get a dopamine bump while meeting your daily dose of exercise—a recent study found that the calorie burn you get from many of the Wii Fit Plus and Wii Sports games count as moderate-intensity exercise.[40] Another study found that both Step and Hula games on Wii Fit burn calories equal to walking at a 3.5-mile-per-hour pace. Because Hula involves your whole body, researchers said, at the intermediate level you can burn 5 calories per minute.[41]

And before you knock video games as mindless, listen up: Research has shown video game playing to improve attention span, motor and visual skills, and cognition and short-term memory—all brain builders.[42] In fact, video games have been used to train pilots on tricky landings and to help rehabilitate the entire nervous system of stroke patients. Just limit your nonexercise video game playing to an hour or less at a time.

Cool down for better sleep. We know that a good night's sleep is indispensable for your PFC to be on top of its game. Basic sleep hygiene—keep lights low, TV off, stick to a bedtime and wake-up time—will go a long way toward getting you the sleep you need, but here's an unusual trick you can try when you need some extra help: Keep a cool head, literally. In a small study done in 2011, researchers had volunteers try to sleep while wearing a special cap filled with cold water to cool down the frontal cortex of the brain.[43] When using the cap, people with insomnia fell asleep as quickly and stayed asleep for as long as people who didn't have insomnia. More research is needed, but this could lead to important nondrug therapies to help people sleep.

In the meantime, you can try cooling down your pillow with an ice or gel pack before bed, lowering the thermostat in the bedroom, or taking a cool (not cold) shower before you hit the sack. Getting good sleep will strengthen your PFC for the next day's challenges; sufficient sleep also lowers your risk of hypertension, depression, weight gain, and even cancer.

It's time to get up and start your practice. Keep these wise words in mind, by Chris Bradford in *Young Samurai: The Way of the Warrior*: "Tomorrow's victory is today's practice."

CHAPTER 7

Stage 3: Master Recovery

THE MASTER IS THE ONE WHO STAYS ON THE PATH
DAY AFTER DAY, YEAR AFTER YEAR. THE MASTER IS
THE ONE WHO IS WILLING TO TRY, AND FAIL,
AND TRY AGAIN, FOR AS LONG AS HE OR SHE LIVES.
—GEORGE LEONARD, *MASTERY*

Length of Time: The rest of your life

Master Recovery Reward: Maintain/further refine Hunger Fix body composition goal; heighten vigilance and resistance to False Fixes and False Fix lifestyle habits; under stress, refine ability to regroup using Stages 1 and 2 as necessary; become more fearless in the face of adversity; experience higher levels of joy and satisfaction; deepen your sense of spirituality and meaning in life; look and feel your best!

YO-YO MA ON THE CELLO. MARTINA NAVRATILOVA on the tennis court. Plácido Domingo at Carnegie Hall. Georgia O'Keeffe with paintbrush in hand. Tom Brady in the Super Bowl. These folks have distinguished themselves as masters at their craft. They know the secret—that the path to mastery is paved with daily practice. Stage 3 is about *mastery*. That's such a rich and riveting word.

I will never forget a story I heard about three-time Olympian and gold medal–winning gymnast Dominique Dawes, whose gymnastics club is not too far from my home in Maryland. A reporter from the *Washington Post* had come to the facility to observe Dawes training in preparation for the Olympics. That year, the competition was heated as the Americans kept pace with the mission-impossible routines constantly being churned out by the Romanians. As the *Post* reporter sat attentively, Dawes walked to the chalk tray, rubbed her hands, and while gazing at the vault, plotted her complicated dismount. Standing at the end of the carpeted runway, she took a breath, broke into a run, hurdled on the springboard, and sprung onto the vault. Within seconds, she had performed the most difficult dismount designed for female gymnasts. And she nailed it *perfectly*.

Jumping out of his seat, the reporter ran to congratulate her, exclaiming, "You did it! Now we'll win for sure!" Smiling, she politely thanked him and then quietly made her way back to the chalk tray. Puzzled, the reporter asked what she was doing. She replied, "That vault you saw was the first of a thousand I will do."

With mastery comes the humility of knowing that being a master is ephemeral and that the skills will disappear without practice.

In Stage 2, you learned the value of practice. You also saw that your Hunger Fix practice does not have to be an onerous process. Practicing daily meditation, deepening relationships with family and friends, building your new Healthy Fix tribal member support systems, and savoring delicious nourishment and joyful physical activity (crank up that iPod!), you realized that you could feel pleasure and reward without resorting to False Fixes. Fueled with the energy and vitality that comes with your Stage 2: Beginner Recovery accomplishments, it's easier to face off with your addictive urges and to finally acknowledge what an authentic, life-giving reward is: You hunger for fun and fulfillment.

As aikido master and philosopher George Leonard said so well, a master "should understand the joy of it, the fun of it. Being willing to see just how far you can go is the self-surpassing quality that we human beings are stuck with. Evolution is a whole long story of mastery."[1]

So, congratulations on one giant step in your own evolution. You've reached Stage 3. As a Hunger Fix master, you've shed both mental as well as physical weight. You've removed at least 80 percent of your excess body weight, dropped your body fat percentage, lost inches, and maintained or even improved on this achievement for 6 months. In Stage 3, you can continue to shed more of your weight if necessary (mental as well as physical). The key difference is that you'll struggle less. Your brain is bigger and stronger along with your body—recall the Hunger Fix motto, Big Brain, Small Waist—and you have a more dominant amount of mental and physical power to sustain your Hunger Fix lifestyle. You've earned the right to enter Stage 3 and celebrate the beginning of your Master Recovery.

Stage 3 is special. Through dedicated practice, your brain has taken your new Healthy Fix habits and has integrated them into your subconscious. You know you're hooked on authentic rewards when your Healthy Fixes become the knee-jerk go-to response to stresses in life. They have gone from a conscious action requiring vigilance and mindfulness, to one that is so well integrated that it becomes unconscious and mindless in a positive way.

By Stage 3, your life has become more Healthy Fix–centric. You get up in the morning, and central to your daily priorities is the need to honor what it will take to maintain your mental, nutritional, and physical fitness. You'll notice that your bitch-moan-whining has fully reversed—you now complain if you *can't* access a great gym while traveling, or if your favorite Healthy Fix food is sold out, or if you can't find a quiet place for your daily meditation. You become so used to cooking a healthy breakfast that it becomes mentally effortless.

You have humbly accepted that this is the way to go and you do it gladly! You've taken the time and lots of practice to help the brain integrate and build the neural pathways to support this new Healthy Fix, and your entire epigenome has been benefiting from this positive cascade of health.

Don't forget: The Hunger Fix is a lifelong recovery process dependent upon optimal PFC function to heighten and strengthen vigilance to stay on track. Your total number of dopamine D2 receptors drops 6 percent every decade of your life after you turn 20. If you don't remain vigilant and keep building up your brain with Healthy Fixes, that decrease in receptors could provoke a backslide.[2] That's why Stage 3 is about how to *sustain* your Master Recovery for life.

Prepare for Lifelong Recovery

First, it's time for a reality check. When you reach Stage 3, you're definitely entitled to feel proud of how far you've come. But as I've said before, you need to stay vigilant. False Fixes can reassert themselves in the blink of an eye if you become too laid back and stop paying attention. Or maybe a major trauma occurs and you are seriously derailed. It happens to all of us, even the masters.

Like Samantha, who, after achieving her Stage 2 goal of 52 pounds, had a setback that was a game changer. She had a major EpiphaME realizing that her addiction, "the beast," was always lurking should she drop her vigilance under fire.

> The beast never went away, it was just hiding, waiting to strike. I was blindsided, and by the time I really consciously realized what was happening, it was too late. A clear consciousness of what was

happening didn't emerge until real physical terror—
I woke up choking, because stomach acid was running up my throat into my mouth from my anxiety.
I had bought bags of candy, intending to make
Christmas cookies for everyone, but suddenly I had
to feed the beast. I hid candy in the freezer, the car,
even wrapped in a sock strategically placed throughout the house. I felt ashamed, tricked, embarrassed,
mortified, and angry. The anger fired me up and
gave me strength to face the beast. I'm nauseous just
admitting my darkest moments of addiction—
my friends, family, and husband would be shocked
to know!

Samantha was smart and enlightened. She fueled herself with
anger and determination and regrouped. She quickly revisited Stage
1: Detox, spent time in Stage 2, shed the 15 pounds she'd regained,
maintained that loss for 6 months, and now has rejoined her fellow
masters in recovery.

Samantha teaches everyone an invaluable lesson: There is no cure.
Expect ongoing regrouping. And there is rewarding and pleasurable
recovery—for life. Vigilance is the key to achieve this priceless goal.

Throughout the Hunger Fix, I've stressed how important it is to
attack your food addiction in a holistic, comprehensive way using the
Mind, Mouth, Muscle template.

When you use a traditional calorie-cutting "diet" alone, your body
cannot adapt and adjust enough to maintain your weight change. A
recent article published in the New England Journal of Medicine
studied dieters who had dropped 10 percent of their weight and
found that a year later, their appetites were as strong as they'd been
when they were on a weight-loss diet. Their levels of the appetite-
suppressing hormones leptin, peptide YY, and cholecystokinin were

I Need a Fix

Turning Adversity into Mastery

I ran the New York City Marathon in 2001, 6 weeks after 9/11. *Prevention* magazine covered me as I ran with a dozen of my Peeke Performers on this incredible and momentous day. Our picture was the centerfold for the January 2002 issue, and I have that photo and my medal framed on my office wall. As I gaze at the picture, I see Karen, with a mile-wide smile, fit, joyful, and a master of recovery. Her rich story will hit home with most of you and help you understand the master's journey.

Over 20 years ago, 5-foot-3-inch Karen weighed more than 200 pounds. She'd been on a roller coaster of significant ups and downs with her weight most of her life. When a marital crisis occurred, she lost her appetite and dropped 80 pounds. But once her postdivorce reality hit, her False Fixes reappeared and she was north of 180 once again. Together, we began to confront issues of insecurity and lack of confidence in her personal life. Meanwhile, paralleling the rough economy, she'd faced abrupt job change-ups multiple times, and with each bump in the road, those False Fixes were waiting for her.

After the last layoff, something changed. Instead of hopping right back into the cesspool of endless interviews and mountains of paperwork, she called a halt to the insanity. She decided, for the first time in her life, to use that summer to take care of herself. Living near a park was her lifeline. Every day she walked among the trees and along the lake, and she meditated and prayed. She drew from deep inside her for the power to detox off her False Fixes while changing her inner dialogue from one of helplessness, hopelessness, and defeat to one of empowerment and focus.

Once again she entered Stage 2, practicing her Healthy Fix habits. Beginning at 180 pounds, she battled with her addictions and self-destructive urges, but drawing on her bond with nature and her meditation, she found it easier. Her persistence and practice paid off when she hit her 80 percent mark at 140 pounds. And she kept at it.

A stress overeater, she was now calmer and less inclined to reach for a False Fix, noting, "I just did my best and stopped freaking out." Within the 6 months after reaching 140, she entered Stage 3: Master Recovery. Elated with her success at maintaining her achievement, she once again called upon her mental and spiritual energy to tackle a new diagnosis of colitis. Adapting and adjusting, she further refined her Healthy Fixes to accommodate her digestive condition. *"In the midst of difficulty lies opportunity,"* she declared and turned her problem into an opportunity to adapt and adjust and further refine her Healthy Fixes.

Her weight eventually dropped to 115 pounds. At 58 years old, armed with mental serenity and a firm, fit body, Karen's spending her life realizing dreams she's hungered to achieve for years, including a new life partner.

all lower; levels of the hunger hormone ghrelin were higher. Blood tests revealed that hormones and other chemical signals that affect appetite seemed to be signaling for them to eat more than they were.[3]

Of course, this is not the whole picture. There's a bright spot from the same *NEJM* article: Pancreatic polypeptide, a gut satiety hormone that's been shown in a small randomized double-blind placebo-controlled study to reduce food consumption by 15 to 25 percent,[4] was higher. The *NEJM* study also didn't address the effects of long-term exercise, while hundreds of other studies have found that consistent physical activity helps reverse insulin and leptin resistance, resetting our body's natural hunger cues and making muscles better able to burn calories rather than storing them. Exercise also influences the body's stem cells to become bone cells instead of fat cells, a switch that boosts our immune system function, increases the oxygen in our blood, and improves our ability to heal from injuries. And don't forget that exercise directly increases the amount of gray matter and the prefrontal connections in our brains, and that beefed-up PFC helps us make better decisions that override those hormone-driven cues.[5]

The bottom line is that you must gradually and methodically work with your thought process, your nutrition, and your physical activity to successfully control your addiction and sustain that success for a lifetime. Use this three-pronged approach, and the beast of food addiction will be much easier to tame long-term.

Reach for Even Higher Highs

The fact that you've maintained your Stage 2 achievement this far is an indication that the way you did it is sustainable for life. Your ability to hold on to your achievement is a huge neon sign that you've strengthened your PFC enough to successfully battle your innate

1. Upon awakening, open your eyes and say in wonderment, "Wow! I'm still here!" You can laugh, because that's part of the magic. Just remember that nothing is guaranteed, not even waking up—so be grateful for that!

2. Before you get up, lie there for a minute or two and go through your list of gratitudes—think of all the relationships with people, amazing experiences, and important things that contribute to your happiness. Zip through that list, smiling away as you recall meeting your best friend for coffee, or walking your dog in the stillness of the morning, or your terrific presentation before an audience, or the fragrant rose-

I Need a Fix

Mastering Meditation— and the Marathon

CNN's award-winning senior political correspondent Candy Crowley is best known for her articulate and balanced commentary. When she began to anchor her new weekly *State of the Union* show in 2010, Crowley's fans noticed something different about her. She'd shed a significant amount of weight. The blogosphere lit up with speculations about how she did it. In an interview with the *Los Angeles Times,* she shared her secret: swimming, walking, running, and working out with a trainer, along with confronting her False Fixes and pitching the junk, choosing whole foods instead. In addition, she added quiet time through Transcendental Meditation. Crowley summed it up by saying, "I feel great physically. I feel really good. I'm lighter now in a lot of ways."

Flash forward to the summer of 2011 when I had the pleasure of sitting with Candy in her backyard close to my home on the outskirts of Washington. A work in progress, she acknowledges the usual slips and slides in her eating and exercise, but there's something different now. Looking serene and happy, Candy shared how the peace and calm she achieves through her meditation have helped her stay the course and regularly regroup as she continues to be challenged by her 24/7 high-profile life. Her new level of self-care practice and mastery has not only helped her make the right choices but has also fueled personal goals she's hungered to attain for a long time—like running a marathon. I promised that when she was ready, I'd lace up my shoes and pound that Marine Corps Marathon pavement along with her, right by her side.

bushes blossoming outside your window. Recall this list throughout the day when life gets funky. It's extraordinary how your gratitudes will help you gain better perspective of what's really important.

3. Next, sit up and meditate and/or pray to center yourself to stay focused and vigilant as you start your day.

4. When you're done, say, "Today I will _____" and then recommit to your healthy fix habits, sticking to your optimal nutrition and physical activity as well as the mental calm and serenity you'll need in the face of daily stresses.

5. Finally, hop out of bed and say, "Bring it on! I'm ready to adapt and adjust all day long!" Sometimes, having a cup of coffee in your hand adds a little vim, vigor, and vitality to your declaration!

Finally, remember to be grateful for all that you have done to attain your new status as a master of recovery.

Get fearfully high. Have you ever wondered what *is* the draw of clinging to the bar in a roller coaster? Grabbing that zip cord and ripping across a valley? Jumping off a high platform in protective gear during a boot camp retreat? Rock climbing up an 80-foot wall? Bungee jumping, skydiving, or zipping down a ski slope? Turns out that while most of the dopamine neurons in the ventral tegmental area of the brain will gush out some dopamine in response to pleasant stimuli, about 25 percent of those neurons release dopamine in response to fear as well.[6] One of the most reliable sources of dopamine is the fear/excitement combo, which also releases norepinephrine that, together with dopamine, enhances your performance, increasing your alertness and sense of well-being, affecting the brain like a potent combo of speed and cocaine. Thriller suspense movies keep you in a state of constant fear and heightened anticipation, and then—eek!—surprise you with ax murderers jumping out of bushes. The result is one big dopamine bath.[7] Tap into the healthy anxiety of racing against a close competitor in your first sprint triathlon or swimming across a lake. The element of "danger" is there—but the exercise makes it a higher high![8]

Live a high life. Recall that the key to success in food addiction recovery is keeping the PFC strong and powerful and optimally capable of helping guide the right decisions. Once you've reached Stage 3, you've been using your Three M's template to strengthen your PFC to continue to avoid those persons, places, and things that trigger your addictive behavior. Now that we know productive fear (will I make it to the finish line of my first 5-K?) can be a Healthy Fix, it's time to revisit the EpiphaME chart from Chapter 4 and tackle a personal challenge or stress that you've dreamed of confronting and overcoming and reap the rewards of your consistent practice of Healthy Fixes.

Maybe you want to give a speech. Get a new job. Leave a relationship. Go to a bar and ask someone out, or put your profile on Match .com. Ask for a raise. Drop the rest of your excess weight. Whatever it is, now is your time. Start by putting that pen to paper:

1. Use the left column of "Your Adapt and Adjust Plan" chart from Stage 2 (see page 139) to list your prior attempts at this goal.

2. Now, list any False Fixes that blew your shot out of the water.

3. Finally, use all the skills you've developed to come up with an alternate set of Healthy Fix strategies that will help you succeed this time. In addition, make a list of all the external resources and support that could help you. The list should have at least 10 alternate Healthy Fix strategies per False Fix that stopped you in the past. You don't have to do all these Healthy Fixes—but these are your rescue plan options.

You may not have attacked these goals due to fear of failure, along with past negative feelings toward yourself. However, since you've achieved Stage 3 status, it's time to rock and roll. Always ask yourself, "What's the worst that could happen?" Then you realize that the consequences are usually not that bad and you can move on if things don't pan out.

Want to ask for that promotion—or are you ready to polish up that résumé and move on to a new career? Check in with your PFC and draw upon your brain's ability to help you plan, strategize, organize, and launch your new initiative. After all, your daily meditation, consistent physical activity, and nourishing foods provide you with the courage and fortitude to take careful risks and live with the consequences, good, bad, or otherwise.

This is your time—you no longer have to live with the frustration, heartache, or self-sabotage that has plagued you for years. You have the ultrabuff brain to do this—and your brain will only get stronger with the challenge. As you peel layers off yourself, you reveal the real you to the world—it's scary but, thanks to dopamine, always exhilarating!

You're higher when you refire. The bigger the fear and excitement, the bigger the rush.[9] Innovation and creativity, entrepreneurship, risk taking—all are big dopamine boosters. As your brain switches from short-term focus to a longer horizon, you can tackle that BIG dream, the one that really scares and excites you. The one that whispers, *I coulda been a contender.*

News flash: You already are. And now it's time to show the rest of the world your rock-star self.

Answer the question: What would you do if you felt absolutely no fear and had limitless time and money? Would you create art? Start your own business? Try out for a play? Learn to pole dance? Run for political office?

To extend your Hunger Fix program into the rest of your life, your assignment is to find an ongoing interest or endeavor that gives your life meaning. Longer-lasting, sometimes frustrating tasks that you love actually yield more rewards and extend your life longer than a series of quick hits of happiness, even if they're more challenging on the day-to-day level.

This is part of the reason why retiring early doesn't necessarily extend your life. For that matter, I never use the word *retire*. Like my good friend and colleague Ken Cooper, MD, founder of the Cooper Institute, says, Don't retire, *refire!* That means you reinvent yourself countless times in your lifetime. Never, ever stop growing. Just keep refiring.

People need purpose. While you may feel like "balance" is an elusive goal—what the heck does that word mean, anyway?—when you're busy with work, family, home, and volunteering in your community, and you have a lot of people who need you, that constant challenge can be good and pleasurable for you. In the recent book *The Longevity Project,* authors Howard S. Friedman and Leslie R. Martin point to the research that says the people who live longest are "those who were most engaged in pursuing their goals."

Wonder if your current interest could hold you long-term? Consider these characteristics common to all high-quality endeavors of long-term interest. Does it:

- Engage and satisfy your curiosity?
- Help you feel wonder and excitement?
- Feel effortlessly interesting and engaging (i.e., you don't have to force yourself to do it)?
- Offer you a sense of total absorption and interest—a feeling of flow, of being in the moment?
- Feel safe?
- Challenge you?
- Spark moments of novelty, change, mystery, and/or a sense of possibility?
- Feel important to you?
- Require effort and attention?
- Stimulate you to consider alternate viewpoints and remain open to changing your mind?

According to researchers at the University of California, Santa Barbara, interests like this are what shape the world:

> Interest is the primary instigator of personal growth, creative endeavor, and development of intelligence. Interest, then, not only broadens an individual's

momentary thought-action repertoire as the individual
is enticed to explore, but over time and as a product of
sustained exploration, interest also builds the individual's store of knowledge and cognitive abilities. Again,
these become durable resources that can be accessed
in later moments, and in other emotional states.[10]

It's time to live your dreams.

Tap into the helper's high. Want to really stir up that dopamine and
keep your False Fixes reined in? Turn your energies outward to others.
As a relatively recent convert to the Healthy Fix lifestyle, you are still
close enough to identify with the fears and obstacles that held you back
in the past. Use this compassion and empathy to help others who are
scared and just beginning their path. Adopt the credo of learning doctors: See one, do one, teach one. Consider becoming a personal trainer,
a coach, a yoga teacher, a Big Brother or Sister. Do you know how
many fitness professionals were once overweight or obese? A truck-
load. They're no fools. They get the win-win of staying in shape and
sharing the message simultaneously. Those Weight Watchers leaders
have been there and done that and are now helping to mentor others.

Perhaps become a crisis counselor or work at a battered women's
shelter. The point is to get out of yourself and into helping others.
Share the wealth of your new Hunger Fix lifestyle. Anything you can
do to help other people who've struggled with your same or similar
demons will protect your own recovery. Case Western researchers
found that alcoholics who helped others in their recovery—as "spon-
sors" or other mentors—were twice as successful at staying clean as
those who did not help others. And a staggering 94 percent of those
who do help others experience lower levels of depression.[11]

Not only will the practice reinforce the good you've done, you'll get
ready access to the helper's high, a well-proven Healthy Fix. One NIH
bran scan study found that when people simply thought of donating

money to help other people, their dopamine reward system lights up.[12] Imagine what happens when you volunteer on a regular basis.

To keep your own motivation for your Healthy Fix lifestyle up, consider working with kids to get them active. Because their brains are still developing, kids are more vulnerable to False Fixes. The prevalence of obesity among US children between ages 6 and 11 has tripled, increasing from 6.5 percent in 1980 to 19.6 percent in 2008—an even steeper trajectory than in adults. If the same addictive brain changes are taking place in these kids as they're growing, what kinds of chances will they have to ever kick their False Fixes? We have to do what we can to catch them before they get False Fixed so we don't pass along this problem to future generations.

Obese kids spend 2 hours a day in front of the TV or computer. They don't exercise as frequently, take gym class, or join a sports team as often as normal-weight kids.[13] Look into your local school or youth sports organization to see if they need volunteers—they *always* need volunteers. Or start an after-school running program, such as Girls on the Run (www.girlsontherun.org). Everybody wins.

Broaden your tribe. In Stage 2 you began to create a new tribe of people who support you on your Healthy Fix journey. Don't stop adding more tribal members. Everywhere you go, keep your ears and eyes open for exciting, challenging, interesting folks with other points of view, preferences, experiences—and all that variety will delight your reward system while it challenges your brain to work a bit harder without you even realizing it. Because all those friends will have a broader range of interests, you'll gain access to a more expansive repertoire of activities as well. One study found that those people who had a wider network of friends had a genetic propensity for novelty seeking. As adults, those people showed more flexible thinking. So clearly, it's in your DNA—embrace a lot of friendships![14] Studies consistently find that people with a wide circle of friends enjoy a significantly increased quality of life and longer health span.

Share your highs for science. We talked about the successful losers in Stage 2, the members of the National Weight Control Registry. Well, addicts have their own registry: the National Quit & Recovery Registry (www.quitandrecovery.org). Scientists from Virginia Tech Carilion Research Institute have gathered the experiences of people

I Need a Fix

The Making of a Teenage Master

Fifteen-year-old Hillary (aka Hilly) marched into my office, planted herself in the chair in front of my desk, and declared, "I am *not* going to college looking and feeling the way I do. I want to change, and I'm ready." Haunted by her family's obesity genes, Hilly was obese most of her young life. By the time she was 13, her 5-foot-11 frame was carrying almost 300 pounds. Her EpiphaME occurred when kids teased her at her own bat mitzvah.

Mustering up all of the adolescent courage and fortitude she could find, she pushed forward with her Healthy Fix plan. Detox was not easy, given that she was a teen surrounded by wall-to-wall snacking and parties as well as by close family members still battling their own food addictions. But she hung in there.

Then a funny thing happened once she reached about 210 pounds. She stopped. Puzzled, I asked her what was up. Together we dug up a traumatic memory that had deeply affected her: When she was a preteen, her parents had taken her to a weight-management specialist, a physician who, upon meeting Hilly, declared that she would probably never see the other side of 200. He wore a white coat. She believed him. I told her he made a terrible mistake and to completely disregard that statement.

It took a while, but eventually she crept toward 200 and finally, one glorious spring day, over the threshold she went. College was a land mine of challenges, all of which she navigated, emerging a bright and highly accomplished PR professional by day. And comic by night.

Yep, Hilly's a talented stand-up comedian, and she's used this unique skill to help others with weight issues. Nothing is sacred, from Oprah's travails to weight-obsessed young adults her age. ("I'm so proud of myself. I've started to take a yogalates class—I do Pilates while eating frozen yogurt.") People relate to and love her message, because she speaks as a master. The laughter and joy give her a helper's high while powering her continued work through myriad issues related to her own weight journey.

Even after 17 years, she's still learning and practicing. After entering into a special relationship, she did as most women do—she gained a few pounds. She's adapting and adjusting, learning how to integrate her guy into her Hunger Fix lifestyle. Like a true master.

who've struggled with tobacco, alcohol, drugs, gambling, sex addiction—and food addiction. "Recovery heroes" share their insights with the objective of helping addicts and researchers alike. Dr. Nora Volkow is hoping that the launch of the registry will decrease the stigma of addiction, help people draw inspiration from each other, and shift researchers' focus away from detox to where the real work of beating an addiction truly lies: recovery. So log on and sign up today.

Memorize your high. Just the act of picking up a book, opening the

I Need a Fix

Done with Numb

A strong family history for addiction was drilled into Meredith's epigenome, and all it took was her parents' divorce to activate those vulnerable genes. Overeating, drinking alcohol to excess, chasing guys, and spending too much money—Meredith was drowning in her cross-addictions, doing anything to numb the pain. But nothing could dull the anguish or quiet the voices of self-destruction until she discovered her own healthy voice.

It was a pleasure to be part of Meredith's remarkable journey as she underwent detox and began a lifetime of recovery. She has shed the physical weight along with immeasurable mental weight and has channeled her energy into regular exercise, spirituality, and multimedia messaging to support others who share her addictions. As she put it, "I found out in treatment that this disease I had wasn't about the food or any other substance or behavior I engaged in when I was giving it power. It was about how those things made me feel. *It was about the fix they gave me.* It was about that high that would take me away from whatever was bothering me in the moment. Whether it was food, alcohol, shopping, horoscopes, or men—I tried to stuff myself, numb myself, and run away from myself." No more. Meredith is now a leading voice in the food addiction and recovery movement. Founder of the Healthy Voice (www.healthyvoice.org), she shares her mastery and humanity with so many who are still confused, distraught, and in the grips of their addictions, the False Fixes. To them she says, "I see people giving power to the sugar, letting it run their lives. I've seen people I love go through it. I've seen myself go through it. I do *not* want to give that stuff power in my toughest moments." Spoken like a true master.

Appreciate the Benefits of Your Unique Brain

While you may have struggled for years with the effects of your depleted dopamine receptors, recent research suggests there was a silver lining. *Scientific American Mind* reported on researchers at the Karolinska Institute in Stockholm, Sweden, who used brain scans to look at the D2 receptors in the brains of some of the most creative people. Turns out that the lower density of D2 receptors results in less cognitive "filtering" of incoming information—which actually leads people to think more creatively.

Other scientists have found similar links between addicts' penchant for taking risks and compulsive need for novelty and the mark of transformational leaders. High-functioning executives often share the same catch-22 that plagues food addicts: They crave more stimulation but feel it less—so they're driven to accomplish greater and greater goals to feel that high. The only difference between a cocaine addict one line from OD and a visionary leader with a drive to succeed is the self-regulation necessary to harness and master that drive—which is why you've been doing your PFC training.

While your genes may have given you quite a struggle in the past, take a moment to appreciate the whole picture. Your most dearly beloved hobbies and interests may have sprung from the very genes that predisposed you for food addiction—and now's the time to make the most of them. Onward![15]

---

cover, and starting to read can increase the concentration of dopamine in your brain. If you keep challenging yourself—say, with a intense word-association game—you'll get an increase of dopamine in the areas of your brain associated with learning and memory, particularly those that involve associations between novel stimuli and rewards.[16] Researchers from Sweden have proved that even silly memory games that require you to parrot back strings of eight numbers can physically change the number of dopamine receptors in your brain. The scientists had participants do these exercises for 30 minutes a day, five times a week for 5 weeks. The types of changes they saw could enhance your own working memory, the ability to remember what you're going to do next or help you keep information in your mind while you make decisions—critical skills that are lacking in people with ADHD and age-related cognitive decline.[17]

Clean up persons, places, and things in your life to keep the high going. Starting with the Detox stage, we've made it clear that you need to keep examining the persons, places, and things in your life to see if they support your Healthy Fix lifestyle. This means taking a cold, hard look at your whole living and working environment, continuing to refine it to optimize your long-term success. This is tough stuff to face and implement, but it's mandatory if you're going to head down the path to mastery.

We often use the fog of False Fixes to mask the pain we feel about certain persons, places, and things in our lives that we *know* are impeding our ability to achieve our healthiest lifestyle. You may have never felt as strong as you do right now, so if you have not done so earlier in the Hunger Fix program, now is the time that you must come face-to-face with these realities and develop the courage and fortitude to manage them. I call it "relationship creation, elimination, or modification." Scary, I know. This is a deal breaker for so many people. To decide to leave a relationship, job, or hometown requires a strong support system.

Go back to your video or written journal from Stages 1 and 2 and watch the progression, in order. Watch your physical body change as the light within you starts to glow brighter. Read the journal pages you wrote about your Healthy Hunger—what pieces of your Healthy Hunger have you already realized? Which ones have you not? What is standing in your way? Now is the time to face up to those fears.

If you need help, reach out—a therapist can guide you through a rough transition. The talking you do with a talented psychologist or counselor actually helps change the neuronal structure of your brain. In discussing your deepest fears, you with the assistance of your doctor can reframe old issues that may be blocking your ability to be successful, but in a safe environment so you can develop healthier ways of coping and reacting.

Stage 3: Mouth

By now, your body has access to so many Healthy Fixes that you can broaden your focus from some of the more protein-rich dopamine-boosting foods to foods that support the optimal health of your epigenome—overall, a more antioxidant-rich, high-quality protein and vegetable-based diet. The beautiful part of this plan is that it's all you need to have a nutritionally optimal diet for life. Your Stage 3 eating plan will have you sampling liberally from foods in all of these categories.

Going further in the spirit of challenging yourself, Stage 3: Mouth is all about expanding and deepening your relationship with food. Now that you've gotten beyond mere survival, it's time to find a more nuanced, more meaningful reward from food. You are literally going to get your hands dirty.

You will deepen your appreciation for dopamine-boosting, genetically healthy foods that support overall wellness by growing, preparing, and sharing Healthy Fix Foods with others. The challenge of learning new skills like creative cooking stimulates neurogenesis and heightens enjoyment while it also highlights how far you have come from the self-destructive false rewards of low-quality, toxic False Fix foods.

Try to cook whenever you can. Cooking helps you redefine your relationship with food, which has probably been conflicted at best during your active periods of food addiction. Cooking is an essential part of the healing process. Nothing fancy is required—just an appreciation of the "safe" foods that will keep cravings at bay (and taste delicious and satisfying). In Detox, your food fear was at its height. In Stage 3, you've forged a new relationship with food through persistent practices. Cooking allows the food addict in you to fall in love with whole foods and crave the right fix.

Double-down on the Hunger Fix food plan to make positive

epigenetic changes. A fascinating example of how a diet similar to the Hunger Fix eating plan tilts the epigenetic equation in your favor was demonstrated by researchers in Norway. Their study, published in 2011, examined the effects of diet on gene expression. They had volunteers switch between a strict diet that provided 65 percent of its calories from carbohydrates and one similar to the Hunger Fix macronutrient mix, with its equal proportions of carbs, protein, and fat. Blood tests were used to compare gene activity for each person while on each diet. The higher-carb diet, especially refined carbs, caused certain genes to, in the words of the lead researcher "work overtime." Some of those genes were involved in causing metabolic inflammation, a state of heightened immune system alertness that contributes to the risk of many chronic illnesses. Other genes were known to raise the risk of cardiovascular disease, diabetes, certain types of cancer, and even dementia.[18]

Notably, the diets used in the study were individualized for each person so that they wouldn't cause weight gain. Which means that even if you're not taking in too many calories, a diet with too many carbs could be putting you at risk by activating unhealthy genes.

Get "prudent" about your diet. Even if you don't always drop your carb intake as low as 30 percent, easing off processed and refined carbs helps protect you from insulin resistance, that bad-news condition that's linked to epigenetically driven diabetes, heart disease, and cancer, not to mention cognitive decline, neurological damage, and runaway hunger. One study, which drew from an international project called INTERHEART that collected heart disease data from 27,000 people in 52 countries around the world, found evidence that people who eat lots of whole vegetables and fruits actually eliminated the effects of a specific gene, 9p21, the variants of which are known to raise heart disease risk. In that study, the researchers identified what they called a prudent diet that lowered heart disease risk: high in raw vegetables, fruits, leafy green vegetables, berries, and nuts.[19] The more that people in the study adhered to that type of diet, the less effect the high-risk gene had. Try these Healthy Fix recipes to move your own diet in a "prudent" direction:

Roasted Beets (page 268)

Asian slaw (page 272)

Italian Farro Salad (page 279)

Broccoli with Garlic and Ginger (page 286)

Kale Chips (page 300)

Berry Yogurt Frozen Ice Pops (page 302)

Snack ideas: small apple or banana with 1 tablespoon peanut butter; 3 dried plums; 1 cup nuts (peanuts, almonds, pistachios, cashews, pecans, walnuts); fruit smoothie (8 ounces soy milk, ½ cup fruit, 1–2 teaspoons chia seeds or flaxseeds, 1 tablespoon oat bran)

Incorporate more methyl donor and other epigenetic-positive foods. Your genes don't know it, but their neighborhood's going to continue to undergo some serious renovation in Stage 3. To make the positive epigenetic changes that will turn on healthy genes, you'll need to keep your body supplied with the methyl groups that flip the switches. Those methyl groups are molecules that get physically attached to your DNA to partially or completely block certain genes from being expressed, so you don't want to run out of them. Be sure your everyday diet includes lots of these methyl-friendly nutrients.[20, 21]

Betaine breaks down the toxic by-products of SAM synthesis. (S-adenosylmethionine, or SAM, is present in most body tissues and fluids, supporting the immune system and cell membranes and helping with production of neurotransmitters such as serotonin, melatonin, and dopamine.[22]) Betaine also helps the liver process fats and reduces the levels of dangerous homocysteine in the blood.[23] *Good sources include* wheat, whole wheat bread, spinach, shellfish, and sugar beets (iced tea is a moderate source).

Butyrate increases histone acetylation, turning on health-protective genes, which may increase life span. Butyrate also increases the number of neurons in the GI tract, helping increase digestive health. *Good sources include* all fiber foods, especially oat bran and apple pectin (butyrate is produced as a by-product of the fiber fermentation process in the intestines).

Choline is a methyl donor to SAM, influencing DNA and histone methylation, two central epigenomic processes that regulate gene expression.[24] As we mentioned in Chapter 6, choline is also a precursor to acetylcholine, a neurotransmitter that supports good memory and muscle control.[25] *Good sources include* chicken, egg yolks, beef, turkey, wheat germ, cod, brussels sprouts, broccoli, shrimp, salmon, fat-free milk, peanut butter.

Diallyl disulphide (DADS) increases histone acetylation, which turns on anticancer genes. *Good sources include* garlic, shallots, onions, chives.[26]

Folate synthesizes methionine. *Good sources include* romaine, black-eyed peas, spinach, turnip greens, collard greens, mustard greens, asparagus, beets, cauliflower, broccoli, summer squash, cabbage, lentils, bell peppers, pinto beans, papaya.

Genistein increases methylation and prevents cancer through an as-yet unknown mechanism. *Good sources include* soy and soy products, fava beans, kudzu, and coffee.

Methionine synthesizes SAM. *Good sources include* eggs, sesame seeds, Brazil nuts, fish, peppers, spinach.

Resveratrol removes acetyl groups from histones, improving health (shown in lab mice). *Good sources include* red wine, grapes, grape juice, peanuts, blueberries, and cranberries.[27]

Sulforaphane increases histone acetylation, which turns on on anti-cancer genes. *Good sources include* broccoli, brussels sprouts, cabbage.

Vitamin B$_{12}$ works with folic acid, helping to synthesize DNA. *Good sources include* sardines, salmon, venison, shellfish (clams are the best source), lamb, milk, cod.

Vitamin B$_6$ synthesizes methionine. *Good sources include* chickpeas (also a great source of tryptophan, a precursor of serotonin), yellowfin tuna, salmon, roast chicken breast, bananas, turkey, marinara sauce.[28]

Season with secret weapons. Becoming adept at preparing different kinds of meals helps you appreciate food as more than a source of quick gustatory pleasure; the satisfaction you get from being a skilled cook is a powerful Healthy Fix. Whatever types of cuisine you choose to prepare, try incorporating these secret food weapons suggested by food scientist and author Steven A. Witherly, PhD.[29] These tricks are well known to the food industry—Witherly has worked at Carnation and Nestlé, among other places—but they can also be used benignly by professional chefs and home cooks to add flavor and complexity to all sorts of Healthy Fix recipes. And if you cook for friends or family, these tactics will put to rest the myth that healthy food can't taste great. (See Witherly's book, *Why Humans Like Junk Food*, for his full list of "secret-weapon pleasure foods"—a fascinating look into the food industry's secret weapons!)

Soy sauce adds color, richness, and depth of flavor to meats and savory dishes. It's a source of the so-called fifth flavor, umami, which is the sort of savory flavor found in meat but also in tomatoes, cheese, and mushrooms. Try soy sauce in sauces, stews, bean dishes, or Caesar salad. Used sparingly, it can even wake up the flavor of sweet baked goods and chocolate desserts. Since soy sauce is notoriously salty, be sure to check the overall salt content of your recipes. Reduced-sodium soy sauces can work just as well.

Garlic increases the flavor of savory foods and stimulates multiple taste systems in the mouth. Plus it's been linked to improved immunity, better cholesterol profiles, and other health benefits. If you have doubts about garlic's pungent flavor, start by roasting it (drizzle two bulbs with olive oil, place in a baking dish, cover with foil, and roast in the oven at 400 degrees until soft and golden, about an hour). You can squeeze the softened garlic into or onto almost anything (try it on bread or potatoes); the flavor becomes mellow and creamy.

Shallots are found in most professional kitchens because they add a distinct flavor to many dishes, from stews to spring rolls. Shallots share many of the health-boosting phytochemicals of garlic and onions but don't give you bad breath. Try using them with, or in place, of onions when making soups, sauces, or stir-fries.

Spice blends, like Emeril Lagasse's famous Essence, are a quick way to enhance the pleasure and flavor of food. There are countless options on the market; have fun experimenting to find the ones you like best. You can also make your own blends with dried or fresh spices. Hot spices like chili powder can stimulate the release of endorphins like serotonin. Nutmeg inhibits the breakdown of dopamine. One study found that curcumin produced epigenetic changes that suppressed tumor growth in colon cancer cells.[30]

Ban the can, for good. I hope you've been trying to reduce your dependency on canned foods. If so, you've helped your body avoid what may prove to be one of the most common triggers for epigenetically modulated obesity: Biphenol A, which we talked about in Chapter 4, lines almost every single can of food produced in America. BPA is also found in plastics labeled with a 3 or 7. (Containers labeled with a 1, 2, 4, 5, and 6 are very unlikely to have BPA.) Lab studies have found that rats' exposure to BPA can reduce DNA methylation of a gene linked to obesity by up to 31 percent. If these results prove similar in humans, some researchers suspect we may have found another one of the causes for the exploding obesity epidemic.[31] (Note that a diet that included genistein, a component of soy products, helped lessen this effect. See page 185 for more info on methyl donor foods.)

Connect with food on another level. Now that you've gotten beyond mere survival, it's time to find a more nuanced, more meaningful reward from food. Take an interest in where your food comes from. Go to your local farmers' market to actually meet the people who grow your food and raise your meat. Learn about what's available in your neighborhood. Commit to buying things produced within 100 miles of your house. You're getting a healthy high right off the land! This deeper sense of responsibility for where your food comes from can only increase your appreciation for your surrounding community and enhance your connections—not to mention get you much fresher, tastier food!

Take a gourmet cooking class. Once you've started to taste the difference between locally grown produce and the tasteless cardboard shipped in from Latin America, you may be inspired to cook more. Go deep into that interest—take a gourmet cooking class. Learn to taste and savor, to relish every bite, and to turn meal preparation and eating into a downright sensual experience. It's a cooking high! Not only will you learn how to make food taste amazing without adding tons of extra fat and salt, you'll engage your brain in an intellectual and creative pursuit that has no limits—zero! You could learn something new about the artful preparation of food every day for the rest of your life.

Dig in. Create a backyard vegetable garden or, if you're an urban dweller, find where community plots are offered. There is simply nothing like eating a tomato that's still warm from the sun and has the scent of the vine on its skin. If you have the space and means, consider building a chicken coop in your backyard for a fresh omega-3-rich egg supply for just pennies a day! With each one of these steps, you're intensifying the dopamine blast from the sensual pleasure of food with the added brain-enhancing benefits of continued creative exploration.

Find another comfort. Most of you have used food for comfort. False Fixes were usually the go-to way to mend a broken heart, numb the pain of loneliness, or angrily rebel against a world that doesn't understand you. You used to be hungry for the fix you got from them. They were your anesthetic. No more. But just to be safe, do this simple exercise—as a master of recovery you should breeze right through.

1. List all of the False Fixes you relied on as comfort foods.

2. For each item, name at least two Healthy Fixes that you would now do in place of the False Fix. For example, instead of diving into a gallon of Ben & Jerry's when your presentation at work didn't go so well, you can call a friend for support and understanding, make an appointment with your boss for a productive discussion about what happened, take a walk, or hit the gym and beat the living crap out of the punching bag/treadmill/elliptical/spin bike.

3. Proactively look ahead at your schedule this week. Identify events, people, places, and things that may be challenging and potentially kick you into a greater vulnerability to False Fixes. Create at two possible Healthy Fixes you can rely upon as your plan A and plan B should stress occur.

The bottom line is to be prepared to comfort yourself every day of your life, the Healthy Fix way.

Try some controlled "exposure" experimenting. Is it ever possible to reintroduce a False Fix in a controlled way and not reawaken your addiction and set you down the slippery slope of out of control eating and weight gain? The answer is yes, but with a few cautionary caveats.

As you know by now, there is a wide spectrum of food addiction. What I have observed over the years is that it is indeed possible for some people to reintroduce controlled amounts of their previous False Fixes, while other folks must maintain abstinence for life. This is treacherous territory, so tread carefully. *When in doubt, bag it and don't tempt fate.* I do not recommend a controlled exposure experiment if you:

1. Have cross-addictions (food addiction plus any combination of other addictions including alcohol, drugs, cigarettes, sex, gambling, shopping) and/or a strong history of cross-addictions in your direct family line.

2. Have a history of compulsive overeating resulting in the gain of at least 50 to 100 pounds or more.

3. Have a history of bariatric surgery (with a typical weight removal of 50 to 200 pounds).

4. Attempted to reintroduce a False Fix during a relapse in Detox or Stage 2 and this reexposure led to serious overeating and bingeing and a definite sense of feeling completely out of control.

5. Are under significant psychological and/or physical stress, as this increases your vulnerability to resorting to False Fixes.

6. Have a history of an eating disorder.

7. Have a medical condition (such as diabetes or heart disease) that will be worsened by reintroduction of the False Fix.

8. Have a mental condition that increases your tendency to overeat (such as depression or bipolar disorders).

9. Are on medications associated with appetite stimulation and weight gain.

A reintroduction of a False Fix food is not recommended for anyone with one or any combination of these criteria.

What about everyone else? So long as criteria 1 through 9 above are not applicable, and you've followed the Hunger Fix plan for over 6 months with sustained success, then if you want to experiment, proceed cautiously. If an occasion happens and you are considering reintroducing a False Fix food, plan ahead. Know what you want. Ideally you:

- Are eliminating any junk-food-like products that are completely processed. *Warning:* If you have not eaten refined sugar or fatty/salty foods for a long time, consuming them may lead to a strange taste in your mouth, as the refined sugar food product tastes too sweet and not as rewarding as expected. Also, you may experience GI upset if you overeat any sugary/fatty/salty food product, since your intestines are not prepared to break down the foods appropriately. This is why it's better to stick with small portions of a high-quality treat, not junky refined and processed products. Think twice about what you're putting in your mouth!

- Strive to enjoy the highest quality food treat you can find—a scoop of the best ice cream, one homemade oatmeal cookie, a small slice of birthday cake from the best bakery in town, a small serving of whole wheat or spinach pasta.

The safest way to do the experiment is to:

- Make it crystal clear up front that you want to delight in a high-quality treat for the pure pleasure of savoring the culinary experience.

Eat Twice as Much and Still Lose Weight?

Eating whole foods may help kick False Fixes, for several reasons. A study at Case Western University found when overweight apes were given access to a diet rich in greens such as romaine lettuce, dandelion greens, endive, alfalfa, green beans, a handful of flaxseed, and multivitamins (inside of smushed bananas), they were able to eat twice as many calories as previously yet dropped an average of 65 pounds each. Why? Scientists are not entirely sure—perhaps switching from the bucketfuls of high-sugar/high-starch foods the zoo had used for years to a diet composed mostly of greens had something to do with it. Another major reason may have been the change in their activity level—instead of spending 25 percent of their day eating a hand-delivered diet, the primates now spend two-thirds of their day feeding and foraging for their own foods.[32]

While we'll never be able to duplicate the calorie-burning power of swinging from trees and tearing off branches to nibble on, we might get some of the same benefits from planting and tending our own organic gardens of vegetables—heavy on the greens.[33] Spinach, kale, broccoli, red and green bell peppers, beans—all are easy to plant and tend, and much cheaper from your own garden. Not to mention the brain benefits of being out in green space. Numerous studies have found that time in nature calms the mind, allows us to focus, and even improves mood and self-esteem. A recent UK meta-analysis showed a dose-response relationship for time in nature and better mental health—a pronounced effect showed up even after just 5 minutes outside.[34]

- Never ever try this if you're hungry right before a meal or snack. Ideally you will be eating on a normal schedule, and the "treat" will occur either during or immediately after your normal satisfying protein-fiber-healthy fat meal or snack.
- Do a stress/emotion check and make certain you're not about to engage in a full-out emotionally charged stress-eating binge.
- Order something you will share with one or more persons.
- Consider designating another person as your "chaperone," someone you trust to help you back down, if necessary.
- Use the smallest bowl or plate.
- Choose the smallest (child-size) serving.
- Plan on having a "tasting" of only 1 or 2 spoonfuls or forkfuls.

Once you've taken all these "safety steps," follow this process:

1. Take 1 teaspoonful or forkful and place the food in your mouth. Savor the taste; pay attention to the texture and smell. You are fully aware, awake, engaged, and consciously in the moment, mindful of this mouthful.

2. Stop, put your spoon/fork down, and allow your body to experience this food. Wait 1 minute. Close your eyes and feel your body, sensing either satisfaction and contentment or a loss of control.

3. If you feel as though you are experiencing loss of control and an urge to overeat, the consumption is ended immediately and the experiment comes to an abrupt end. You cannot handle the reintroduction, and you remain abstinent of that food.

4. If you feel satisfied and in control, either stop your tasting there, or take another spoonful/forkful to finish your small serving. In any case, after every taste, put your spoon or fork down and wait for 1 minute. Keep your mind engaged and continue to be vigilant for any sense of losing control.

This is a learning process as you test your options. One woman, Betty Sweeney, learned this lesson the hard way when, after having shed 120 pounds over 2 years, she caved at Christmastime with people badgering her with "For heaven's sake, it's Christmas—time to cele-brate!" and "Come on, it's *just* apple pie." Thinking she could handle it, she ate and completely lost control over the holidays. She quickly revisited Detox, and it took her 3 weeks to get back on track with the help of her trainer, family, and friends. She's been abstinent of those pastries ever since. Live and learn!

If you were able to successfully implement the experiment, and you want to repeat this, be very cautious. A treat is a treat only if it hap-pens occasionally, not every day. Therefore, be strategic, plan ahead, and always be vigilant. Guarantee success by following the directions each time. Be exquisitely aware of your body and mind, scanning for any feelings of loss of control. Remember that most people need to maintain abstinence from their False Fixes. It is only some outliers who can handle reexposure.

One fascinating pilot study on children pointed to the value in learning to "stare down" your False Fixes. An 8-week study of obese 8- to 12-year-olds looked at two groups: One was given appetite awareness training, which trains kids and their parents to recognize true hunger and respond in a healthy way. The other group was trained in cue exposure, which taught the children and their parents strategies to resist cravings for tempting food that was sitting right in front of them. During the study, researchers brought in plates filled with False Fixes and placed them on a table in front of the kids. The kids were then instructed to hold them plates, smell the food, and even take small bites for a period of 20 minutes, while recording the intensity of their cravings—and then they had to throw their beloved food into the garbage can.

After 6 months, the appetite awareness group hadn't really changed their overeating patterns—but the cue exposure group had "signifi-cant" reductions in overeating.[35] That 20-minute stare-down is prob-ably one of the most intense PFC workouts those kids have ever had! But just look what it did for them—and it can work for you, too.

Stage 3: Muscle

Physical activity, as you're now aware, is integral to your life. Instead of numbing yourself with False Fixes, you're medicating with movement. With every step, stretch, swim stroke, cycle spin, hill climb, or weight lifted, you've been powering your brain, reclaiming your reward system, and living your Healthy Fix recovery optimally.

In Stage 3: Master Recovery, you have options. You can keep on with your usual routine, since it's gotten you to Stage 3 successfully. Some of my patients say, "If it ain't broke, don't fix it," and they prefer to keep going with their proven success. That's perfectly fine. Other folks want to challenge themselves further, mixing it up and experimenting more. Stage 3 affords you the opportunity to do that. You now have the success and confidence to push your envelope even further. I encourage my Peeke Performers to get out there and embrace bigger challenges, create new goals, and keep the Healthy Fix recovery robust and alive.

By this point, your exercise habits will have done more than strengthen your body and your mind—they will have significantly elevated your overall self-image. You've stuck with this program for many weeks and months, and you're undoubtedly starting to see serious changes in your body. Maybe it's easier to zip up your pants. Maybe you feel more energy first thing in the morning, and you're bounding out of bed. Maybe you're powering up the stairs without getting winded, or you're running a 10-K this weekend. Whatever signal your body is giving you, know that it is just the beginning of a long life of these kinds of rewards of accomplishment. You know you can achieve your goals, you *know* you can improve and change—because you've done it. Kudos to you!

By this time, you've probably had the "Moving my body every day has to be a part of my life from here until I'm pushing daisies" EpiphaME. In Phase 1: Detox, your body was beginning a long healing process. Racked by food addiction (and perhaps other cross-addictions) and a self-destructive lifestyle centered around scoring your next fix, you had been dissociated from your body and its needs. Working your way through Detox and into Stage 2, you began to experience how feeling better mentally was reinforcing your decisions to become more active, which then supported your mental fitness. You'd birthed a positive lifestyle cycle. You're here at the masters level because you achieved a serious milestone with your mind and body. At least 80 percent of your body weight-loss goal has been achieved. Stage 3 is all about maintaining this grand accomplishment for life.

And moving your body is nonnegotiable if you want to keep the weight off and the food addiction under control.

I Need a Fix

No Excuses

Moving is like breathing. If you can breathe, then you can find some way to move as well. Whenever I sense a patient is resisting exercise, I think of Corina Gutierrez. Corina is a Zumba instructor whom I had the pleasure of meeting when I received the global Zumba International Fitness Mentor Award in 2011 and she was the recipient of a similar award from the Zumba fitness group. I'd expected her to look like a lean, sinewy, muscular dancing machine. Instead I was blown away by a 32-year-old woman in a wheelchair gracefully swaying to the music with her slender upper limbs. Born with osteogenesis imperfecta, she has spent her entire life dealing with extremely fragile bones, bowed legs and arms, kyphosis (a hunched back), and scoliosis (curvature of the spine). As a result, she's been wheelchair bound for years. As a young girl, she experienced more than 200 fractures in her bones. Physicians did not expect her to live beyond the age of 7. Yet she's defied these odds. Here's her secret: Her PFC is bigger than she is. Yep, despite the immense continuing challenges of her life, she keeps smiling. She's a hope generator. She knows her life is limited, but she's making the most of each moment. I wrote about her in my WebMD blog *Everyday Fitness with Pamela Peeke, MD,* and I entitled the essay "Read This the Next Time You Don't Feel Like Getting Active" (http://blogs.webmd.com/pamela-peeke-md/2011/08/read-this-the-next-time-you-dont-feel-like-getting-active.html). I received countless postings from men and women blown away and inspired by her story. So breathe and move.

Become an adult-onset athlete. One of the greatest pleasures I've had is turning people on to their own athletic potential. That doesn't mean I'm sending folks to an Olympic boot camp. Far from it. I just want you to celebrate the incredible things your marvelous body can now do. And your accomplishment is all relative to your age, gender, body composition, physical strengths and limitations, medical conditions, and innate athletic tendencies.

You've probably already had pleasant surprises along the way. Who knew you could hike, run, cycle, swim, or lift weights the way you do now? Hey, who's that dancin' on the dance floor? Is that you shakin' it in hip-hop class? Bet you never thought you'd survive the lotus position, but you're "om"-ing away on your yoga mat. Talk about a strong core, pulling off a set of hundreds in Pilates. Is that you balancing perfectly on one leg in tai chi class? How does it feel perched at the top of a mountain after a long hike, inhaling the vast panorama that surrounds you?

As Betty, a breast cancer survivor and one of my Peeke Performers once said after hiking with me to the top of Green Mountain in Aspen,

> You know, after hours of marching uphill amongst the most beautiful scenery I've ever laid eyes on and then reaching the top, the last thing on my mind was, "God, I wish my thighs were smaller" or "Man, I wish I could eat a bag of chips." Here, gazing at this view, there's no room for negative voices and there's no better reward than being where I am right now.

As the masters of recovery will tell you, one of the most important secrets to their ongoing success is that they keep the momentum going by constantly creating new challenges. By doing so, you don't get bored and get stuck in a rut, becoming vulnerable to your False Fixes. Look around you and find a challenge, any challenge, and give it a try.

I Need a Fix

Cheryl Hikes the Canyon

In 2008, accompanied by hike leaders Steve and Toni from my Red Mountain spa in St. Georges, Utah, I led a group of adventuresome Peeke Performers on one of my rim-to-rim hikes of the Grand Canyon. An advanced hike—11 miles down the north rim, 4 miles across the base, and 11 miles up the south rim—it's definitely not for the faint of heart. Cheryl, a competitive and powerful athlete, remained at the head of the pack. But she hadn't always been like that. Born to a family ripe with obesity genes, Cheryl was a tomboy and an athlete, never rail thin, but strong and muscular. She didn't have a major weight problem until a crisis occurred with her one of her children and she abandoned her self-care. Mindless stress overeating for a long period of time unmasked her genetic potential, eventually resulting in a weight gain of 130 pounds on her 5-foot-5-inch frame.

Despite her husband's desperate entreaties and the concerned warnings from her doctor, Cheryl didn't change. Until her EpiphaME. She was to receive a special award and was damned if she was going to wear some sacklike matronly garb when she walked across that stage. A mental click occurred, and she was off and running. First Detox, where she pitched the sweets, and then recovery. A deeply religious woman, she attributed much of her success to consistent prayer and faith, along with the love and support of her boys and husband. Within 2 years she'd removed the 130 pounds and cross-trained in several sports, and she has sustained that accomplishment for the past 6 years. She celebrated her triumph in the Grand Canyon in a very special way.

It was 105 degrees under sunny skies. Once we hit the base, we hiked to Ribbon Falls, where we stopped for lunch. Everyone took turns jumping under the breathtaking falls and enjoying the welcome relief of cool water on sweaty skin. Cheryl was hesitant. She'd always disdained her body, and soaking it meant showing it off, something foreign and scary to her, even after shedding all of the excess weight. Now it was time to shed the mental weight as well. With a bit of prodding and loving support from the group, she hopped under the veil of water—and something magical happened. She jumped up and down like a little girl, twirling and laughing, free to love herself at long last. As Cheryl recalls: "There was comfort and encouragement pushing me forward. I was thinking about all the good things I have done. I felt like all the negative stuff just left me. Emotions, anxiety, fear get me nowhere, but confidence pushes me forward." Call it the ritual cleansing and transformation of the master.

Infect others with your transformation. *"I'll have what she had!"* was the shout heard round the world as Rob Reiner's mother enviously watched Meg Ryan gyrate with joy in her seat at Katz's Deli in the film *When Harry Met Sally.* As you begin your life as a master of recovery, I'll bet there are a slew of people out there—gym members, family, friends, co-workers—who've been silently watching your transformation, wondering what your secret is. Slowly but surely, one or two or more may come up to you asking, "So, how'd you do it?"

Be honest and tell them there's mental and physical work involved, but it's worth every bead of sweat. I love to quote Vince Lombardi: "The only place where success comes before work is in the dictionary." Then, as a master, why not spend a minute and tell them about your Hunger Fix journey. Remember, you're not their therapist, nutritionist, or fitness professional. Instead, simply lead by example and refer folks to the resources you've used along the way. Each individual needs to customize the journey, but you can help point the way.

One of the most frustrating challenges is when you had your EpiphaME and got it and proceeded to Detox and get going on your journey, but your spouse, boyfriend, girlfriend, mom, dad, bro, sis, or best friend is not ready for change. They're still self-destructing, and you have to either live with or be in contact with them on a regular basis. Preaching will get you nowhere. The winning strategy is to quietly practice your Healthy Fix behaviors and experiment by suggesting a walk in the neighborhood, along the beach, or in a park as a nice opportunity to talk and catch up. Getting out and using your body is practicing covert operations, hoping the other person will begin to have an energizing, mind-body wakeup call. As Nietzsche said, "All truly great thoughts are conceived by walking." Keep walking and infecting others with this transformative Healthy Fix.

Kick-ass challenging cardio: Once you're in Stage 3, reconsidering your endurance and cardio, here's a cardio checklist to assess where you stand now and offer options to kick it up another notch:

Bump up your activities of everyday living. All day long, there are endless opportunities to get up and move your body. Carrying groceries, cleaning the car, decluttering the house, scrubbing floors, cooking meals, mowing the lawn, raking leaves, and planting rosebushes all count as invaluable ways to reward yourself with a bigger brain, toned muscles, and a smaller waist. Like pennies in a piggy bank, at the end of the day your reward is a *wealth of health.*

Challenge and cross-train. In Detox, you experienced an amazing awakening. You took it slow and steady as you trained your mind and body to accept physical movement as a critical part of your Detox and recovery from your False Fixes. In Stage 2, you may have bravely ventured beyond your regular routine of walking or running or cycling or swimming or doing the elliptical to experience new ways to move your body. Maybe you took a spin class, learned to hike, started to run, or took up Zumba or ballroom dancing.

In Stage 3, step up the experimentation—your mind and body are ready for it. Get out there and cross-train; schedule a beginner's triathlon. Challenge yourself to do something your food-addicted self would never have the courage to even think about doing. For example, I host my Peeke Week Grand Canyon retreats at the Red Mountain spa in St. Georges, Utah. Many of the men and women who join me are in Stage 3, ready to challenge themselves with the 2-day, 26.2-mile hike. We even made history when my dear friend and colleague US Surgeon General Regina Benjamin, MD, joined us in 2011—we filmed the entire trip, and it's now in the archives at the Department of Health and Human Services.

Get even more intense! Most of you have tried out the Stage 2 high-intensity interval training (HIIT) beginner's tips. So HIIT it some more! The key to maintaining your Stage 3 accomplishment is to continue your baseline cardio and then push yourself further. Just started running in Stage 2 and pulled off your first 5-K? Do another and another and then bump it to a 10-K and a half-marathon, if that works for you. Your body craves intensity. (Forget hanging upside down from a 30-story building in a Navy SEAL boot camp. It might be intense, but it's not really what you're looking for.)

Don't sit on your newly toned laurels. One of the biggest mistakes

I Need a Fix

Debby's Detox Poetry

Debby darted past others as she and her husband sprinted to the finish line of another 10-K. No way this could have happened 5 years and 65-plus pounds ago. Having spent most of her life battling with her body and weight, Debby had finally had it. I guided Debby, an avowed sugar addict, through her Detox and into Recovery. While practicing her new Healthy Fix lifestyle, she rediscovered her love of poetry and documented her journey.

It's hard to fight a sugar craving.
It's even harder to fight a sugar addiction.
The sugar calls to me—
Luring me into a vision of momentary bliss.

All potential aftershocks seem easy to deal with before indulging.
But trust me—the feelings of losing control, missing goals,
Feeling sick and craving more are never worth it.
While it is hard to fight a sugar craving,
And it's even harder to fight a sugar addiction,
I have proven to myself in the trenches, that it is not impossible.

And there is something else I have learned—
That when I care for myself by saying no to sugar,
I am giving myself the sweetest gift of all.

Spoken like a master.

people make is to stop challenging themselves. Let's get it clear. For the rest of your life you will create goal rewards, work hard to achieve them, and then create more again and again. This is critical to your lifelong mental and physical challenge.

To build on gains, add more frequency. As you become more fit,

I Need a Fix

Bob and Sally Get Real

Bob had been a track star in college, but like so many executives, once he hit the ground running with his career and family life, his 5-foot-11 frame shot from 160 to 240 pounds. He spent hours working out but hadn't fully committed to ditching the refined sugars. Although he dropped weight, he couldn't budge below 200 pounds nor shake his ongoing battle with type 2 diabetes.

When we began to work together, Bob had a major EpiphaME: *"You can't exercise your way through a bad diet."* And so began his journey. First, a Detox off the sugars and on to a Recovery program of shorter, more high-intensity interval training that worked around a pair of bad knees. His goal was to reach 185 after having struggled for so many years. To his amazement, he zipped past 185 and achieved 170 pounds, off all diabetic medicines, with a completely normal blood sugar profile. He's maintained this remarkable achievement and is now a master of recovery. His stellar success infected Sally, his wife, who, when we began to team up, was 56, 5 foot 3, and 140.8 pounds with a body fat of 35 percent.

Postmenopausal and wrestling with hot flashes and an expanding belly, Sally was also the owner of her own company. She felt time constrained. We did the "Creating Your Own EpiphaME" exercise (see Chapter 4) to help her prioritize and create the blueprint for her Healthy Fix choices. She joined Bob in detoxing off the False Fixes, and she made time (through better time management and delegation of responsibilities) to do her cardio and begin weight training. As it turns out, she was losing bone, and she was vitamin D deficient as well. Adding vitamin D–rich foods and supplements, along with weight training, halted the bone loss. Within a year, Sally dropped from a size 10 to a 4, her body fat plunged 19 points to 20 percent, and she's down 22 pounds to 119 pounds, a number she hasn't seen in years. The best news is Bob and Sally are there to support each other each and every day. Two masters of recovery who *got it*—together.

your body adjusts to higher levels of intensity. Be sure to keep challenging yourself and commit to exercise five times a week, if you haven't already. One study in the journal *Health Psychology* found that kids who'd done more vigorous exercise—40 minutes or more, five times a week, for 3 months—had a net gain of 3.8 additional IQ points. MRIs showed that the kids' prefrontal cortex—where decision making, planning, social awareness, and complex thought all take place—was growing, presumably strengthening their executive function abilities.[38]

Just as the brain will maintain optimal cortical capacity and size if it's continuously challenged intellectually, the body too will benefit from constant challenges to improve. Make sure you're hitting all five "food groups" of exercise: strength training, cardio, core training, balance, and flexibility. One way to do this is to set yourself a big goal: Sign up for a triathlon or a cross-country skiing trip in Vermont, or plan a major hike/camping trip (I do a rim-to-rim hike of the Grand Canyon every year). Or start a "streak"—a commitment to exercise every day, for at least a little while, and see how long you can hold out. You'll have to chart a plan to get yourself physically ready and follow it day by day, both activities that flex your prefrontal cortex. But the critical piece here is the goal—goal-directed activities elevate dopamine, and the more dopamine you have, the more motivation you have to achieve those goals.

Master the power mind-body. You've been laying down a consistent practice of strength training in Stage 2. In Stage 3 we take this further. You are now keenly aware that you need your body to be strong to:

- Maintain your new body composition and weight for a lifetime.
- Continue to grow more brain neurons to support your Healthy Fix lifestyle.
- Keep you mentally and physically strong and independent and fit to live your dreams.

"Muscles are hard to get and easy to lose. Fat is easy to get and hard to lose," writes Haruki Murakami in his book *What I Talk About When I Talk About Running.*

Next time someone wants to give you something special for your birthday or for the holidays, tell them you want a session or two with a fitness professional. If you haven't already had the chance to work with a trainer, now's the time. If you're treating yourself, scope out the great deals you can get at most health clubs, especially during sales campaigns throughout the year.

There are many ways to strengthen and tone your body that go beyond your home gym or health club. How about:

- Ashtanga or Bikram yoga
- Advanced Pilates with or without reformer
- Martial arts like jujitsu, kung fu, or even mixed martial arts
- TRX suspension training programs
- Boot camps—weekdays or getaways, for specific sports or general conditioning
- Functional training programs—improving strength, core, and balance for better performance in your activities of daily living
- Cardio boxing for endurance and strengthening
- Rock climbing

Throw your body a curveball. Once you've developed a solid basis of fitness and you feel more confident, you can start to shock your body with unexpected demands. In Stage 2, I challenged you to work your way to 10 bent-knee, straight-leg, or off-the-wall push-ups. In Stage 3, if you don't have disabilities, practice doing 10 push-ups twice a week. Remember, you're multitasking by hitting six muscles all at once.

When you're walking on the grass, do a few cartwheels. Jump down from a boulder while on a hike. Race your kid around the block, both of you at your absolute fastest, flat-out sprint. Take the

What Brown Can Do for You

Not all fat is created equal. Recently, researchers have begun to learn more about "brown fat," a fat that actually burns energy instead of storing it the way our regular old white fat does. Brown fat's job is to regulate our body temperature, and some studies have suggested that keeping indoor heat turned down to 60 degrees can increase the body's caloric expenditure by 100 to 200 calories a day, possibly by forcing the body to use that brown fat to warm itself. Researchers at Ohio State University also discovered that when rats were subjected to complex social situations, that challenge somehow stimulated their bodies to convert white fat into brown fat.[36]

Another study, published in the journal *Nature*, found that a hormone called irisin (or PGC1a) is produced in large quantities in the muscles during exercise. Based on lab results, irisin just may have the power to travel deep into our visceral fat and turn this most dangerous white fat into calorie-burning brown fat and help keep blood sugar levels stable, protecting us from insulin resistance and diabetes.[37]

You know what this says to me? The ultimate Stage 3: Muscle challenge just may be a ski vacation with a new love interest! Think about it: complex social situations, cold air, and a serious, challenging physical workout. That brown fat will keep you warm all through après-ski.

---

stairs—all 30 floors of them. These unexpected bouts of exercise keep both your body and your brain guessing—which builds muscle and protects bone while also giving your brain a little dopamine thrill when you nail it.

Dance all night—just once. If you're on vacation and having a blast, don't turn in too early. Just once, see what it's like to stay up to watch the sun rise. It's a rite of passage that has to be experienced at least once—and you could get a big dopamine surge. Researcher speculate that the section of the brain in charge of sleep and wakefulness, the thalamus, produces extra dopamine to combat the urge to fall asleep.[39] Just make sure you have time to take naps the next day—you're going to "come down" and nothing is going to feel as good as those hotel sheets after a late night out on the town. And watch yourself the next day—after this dopamine surge, you'll get a little lull, which can trigger cravings for False Fixes. Stay vigilant and head for Healthy Fixes instead.

Get hooked on extreme sports. Moving into Stage 3 means you're rethinking what exercise is: not just a method for weight loss and fitness, but an opportunity to set and achieve goals and push out of your comfort zone to try new things. You might find yourself tapping into a healthy, satisfying addiction. A study done by researchers in Norway found that compulsive gamblers and skydivers had similar impulsive behavior, and that both seem addicted to thrill seeking.[40] The difference was that skydivers engaged in their sport more rarely and more intensely than the gamblers, who tended to spend hours on end compulsively gambling without feeling any satisfaction.

The researchers wonder if switching to a healthier form of addiction, like extreme sports, could keep problem gamblers from needing to gamble. Maybe skydiving isn't for you (and is it really a sport?), but finding a sports activity that thrills you and keeps you active—moun-

BEWARE! Even Yo-Yo Dieting Itself Is a False Fix!

Because dopamine is the neurotransmitter involved in motivation and achievement, when you reach a goal, you get a flood of dopamine in your brain. So if you've been focused on a "diet" to "lose 10 pounds" and then you get there—what happens? You feel like you've reached the finish line—you got your rush and there's nothing left to delight your dopamine receptors anymore. Then your achievement just becomes same thing, different day—absolute death to a person who's fixated on novelty and impulsive behavior. You got the reward—and now your brain is looking for the next fix. That's why you have to have a plan and give your brain a *new* fix, preferably something with some risk involved, so you can tantalize those dopamine receptors in another way. To be able to sustain lifelong recovery, then, it is essential to continuously generate new goals to generate more dopamine and higher healthy highs!

tain biking, surfing, martial arts, ocean kayaking, street luge, whatever works—might keep your old unhealthy fixes from finding their way back into your life. Certainly you can expect a dopamine rush, your brain will benefit from learning new skills, your body will stay fit, and, depending on the sport, you might gain the stress-busting benefits of spending time outdoors and interacting with a community. Maybe most important, you'll have a ton of fun.

Display your "never again!" photo with pride. By now you probably don't recognize old pictures of yourself. How could the strong and limber body you now possess have ever been so tired and weak and flabby? Before you trash all the photographic evidence, be sure to keep one or two photos around. You never want to "fall asleep at the meal" like that again—and the pictures will help keep you honest.

Take a double-photo picture frame. Pair the worst snapshot with a picture of you now, the Healthy Fix junkie, looking smokin' hot in an outfit you bought to show off your new body.

Really study the two images. Hang the frame up near your elliptical trainer or your yoga mat or the place you stash your sneaks. Every day before you hit the gym, take a moment to study the pictures—notice the difference in your posture, the way you hold yourself, the glow of your skin, the pride on your face. You're still the same lovable, wonderful person. The difference is you're now officially Hunger Fixed from your False Fixes. You earned every bit of this new body.

No False Fix can ever keep you down again.

You are free to choose to live the Hunger Fix lifestyle—*for life.*

A Final Word

Sit quietly for a moment. Close your eyes and breathe deeply. Think about where you were when you began your Hunger Fix journey— desperate and hopeful, sick and tired of your False Fixes, ready to face off with your addictions, praying all the while for relief from the incessant urges to self-destruct. You worked your way through Detox, accumulating little triumphs, and you finally saw the possibility of living without being ensnared by the lies of addiction. In Stage 2: Beginner Recovery, you learned to self-love and support, nurturing yourself through any relapses, experimenting, and creating a new inner dialogue of motivation and inspiration. Patience, perseverance, and persistence paid off with the achievement of your mental and physical goals. As you transition to Stage 3: Master Recovery, you look back proudly on months and years of slugging it out with your False Fixes, experiencing countless EpiphaMEs along the way, and learning to humbly accept the work and vigilance you must practice for the rest of your life. But the new Healthy Fix rewards are so sweet, so powerful, that your daily rituals of mindfulness seem a small price to pay for such continued joy and satisfaction with your life.

Your Hunger Fix journey is so much bigger than your body weight. In order to achieve mastery, you had to have shed *10 times more mental weight than physical.* Yes, the new badge of honor is no longer "How many pounds have you lost?" but "How many months—years!—have you been clean from your False Fixes?" But go beyond this extraordinary achievement to realize what you've really done here. You've substituted the deadly cycle of falling for the False Hunger of your addictions, which sucked the living life out of you, to living your life-giving hunger for achieving countless dreams you so richly deserve to enjoy.

Now open your eyes and see your new world, a total, holistic environment where you choose to live surrounded by Healthy Fixes and by the people, places, and things that support your lifestyle. You're armed with a brain that is sharper, keenly aware of the presence of False Fixes, and ready to lash out with "It's a lie!" when they try to tempt you time and time again. And you understand that although there is no cure, there is the guarantee that you can live the rest of your life as a master in a rejuvenating, renewing, rejoicing recovery.

Spend your life doing this, all of you. As Albert Einstein said, "Only one who devotes himself to a cause with his whole strength and soul can be a true master. For this reason, mastery demands all of a person."

Relish your newly awakened limitless possibilities. Revel in the achievement of your Healthy Hunger. Once you've learned how to break free, you'll see that there is no limit to the realms of your life in which you can live your Healthy Hunger. Use this power, this flexibility, these razor-sharp adapt-and-adjust reflexes to handle just about anything you can imagine. Congratulations. You've gifted yourself with a rich life of endless opportunities to meet any challenge and fulfill limitless dreams. *That's* the true reward you were hungering for.

CHAPTER 8

The Hunger Fix
Eating Plan

TELL ME WHAT YOU EAT, I'LL TELL YOU WHO YOU ARE.
—ANTHELME BRILLAT-SAVARIN

YOU KNOW BY NOW THAT THE NAME OF THE GAME
is confronting the lies of your False Fixes and replacing them
with the authentic reward and pleasure of your Healthy
Fixes. But making these changes, and saying good-bye to your favorite foods, can be a little nerve-racking. You may envision traumatic days and nights of clutching your tummy in fits of withdrawal. But let me assure you that particular slice of hell will happen only if you attempt to go straight from mountains of gooey, cheesy, fatty, sweet False Fixes to a carefully measured ½ cup of steamed asparagus.

No worries. The Hunger Fix will gently guide you through your food addiction withdrawal, feeding you tasty and satisfying food combinations that keep cravings at bay. And remember, you have all of your Mind, Mouth, and Muscle tips, tools, and techniques to support you.

Before I launch into *what* to eat—with descriptions of food preparation, recipes, and food plans—let's make certain you understand some simple basics about *how* to eat. There are three pillars to keep in mind when thinking about consuming food:

Quality. I've been emphasizing natural, whole foods in meals, snacks, and treats. This chapter will guide you through your dopamine-rich choices. The food plans and combinations were deliberately created to provide you with a feeling of satisfaction all day long. Protein and fiber are critical to eliminating the urge to eat False Fixes, so you'll learn how to prioritize protein in your meals throughout the day. Recent research has shown that nutrient mixes, not calorie content, affect powerful hormonal regulation systems in the brain. A recent study in the journal *Neuron* examined the impact of nutrient balance on orexin and hypocretin, brain hormones that regulate energy balance, wakefulness, and reward. When orexin and hypocretin levels are lowered, people can gain weight and develop narcolepsy. The study found that sugar-rich meals suppressed the activities of these critical hormones, while meals rich in proteins, especially "nonessential" amino acids such as tyrosine, stimulated these hormones. The researchers believe diets rich in protein would lead to optimal energy balance—you're less likely to overeat!—and enhance your ability to be alert and focused.[1]

One of the most concentrated sources of tyrosine is the plant algae spirulina—which is why it's included in the dopamine-boosting Green Monster smoothie (see page 249) to help you get this critical nutrient during Detox and beyond.

Quantity. Even if you're eating whole foods, you could still end up overeating. One of my dearest patients was a woman who was doing really well yet was mystified when she began to plateau a bit. When we really scrutinized her eating, the quality of her foods was excellent. However, the quantity was way out of control.

"But I'm having oatmeal for breakfast!" she'd say.

Yes, but she was preparing over a cup of the raw oatmeal and ladling on 6 tablespoons of walnuts and $1\frac{1}{2}$ cups of berries. The large quantities of cereal and the high caloric concentration of the nuts took a Healthy Fix breakfast and inched it very close to False Fix territory.

That's why I advocate reading your food labels to be aware of what a serving size looks like. If you have to practice with a measuring cup to get a sense of what a ½ cup versus a full cup looks like, then have at it—it won't take long until you've internalized that image. When in doubt, always use a smaller plate or bowl. And if you're uncertain how much you've been served of anything, as a rule of thumb, eat only half or two-thirds, but never the whole thing—get used to seeing a third of your plate covered with food when you hand it back to the server for your doggie bag.

Back in Chapter 5, I asked you to experience the sticker shock of how many calories you consumed during a typical addictive binge. I don't want you to be calorie obsessed, but as an exercise, once you choose the Healthy Fix food combos that work for you, simply keep tabs of the general calorie counts that are presented with the recipes. Use WebMD's Food and Fitness Planner to scope out general calorie counts for other basic foods.

If you're a moderately active woman, the general daily range is from 1,200 to 1,600 calories, based on age and activity level. (You'll never go below 1,200 calories.)

If you're a moderately active man of average build, the range is usually 1,600 to 2,000 calories, based on age and activity level. (You'll never go below 1,400 calories.)

Best of all, by calling on your newly empowered prefrontal cortex to help rein in impulses and overeating, you'll learn how to control portions without having to count every single calorie. You'll know the general serving size, eat more slowly, and allow your body to feel satisfied. You'll soon master what the world-renowned Okinawan centenarians have done for years. Prior to every meal, they say, "*Hara hachi bu*," which translated is, "Eat until you're 80 percent full."

Frequency. The timing of your meals and snacks means that you need to understand when you're truly hungry. Most people who have been overeating out of control for the long term are completely confused about body signals. Hunger is a true biological sensation that says you *need* food to survive. Clearly you're rarely in a life-and-death survival scenario when you're hungry, but it's your body simply saying "Hey, time for nourishment."

Appetite, on the other hand, is about what you *want* to eat. This heavily conditioned response is fraught with memories of reward and pleasure. Now, when appetite is working in harmony with hunger, you make magic together. For instance, you wake up in the morning and you're hungry for breakfast. Wandering into the kitchen, your dopamine surges as you smell freshly brewed coffee. Appetite is kicking in. Then you see your options. Wow, that spinach omelet with a bowl of mixed berries is a sweet memory, and as you conjure it, you want it. Off to the omelet pan you go.

The golden rule is to eat roughly every 3 to 4 hours to stave off hunger while controlling appetite and cravings. The classic template is to eat breakfast, a morning snack (only if you finished breakfast by 8:00 and your lunch is 12:00 or 1:00 p.m.), lunch, midafternoon snack, and dinner. Aside from these times, when you have the urge to eat, do a hunger check: Are you truly hungry? Do you feel a rumbling in your stomach? If you are hungry, what is it that you desire—a False Fix or a healthy meal/snack? Trouble occurs when you're not hungry but your appetite is stirred by cues and triggers. Watch out! This is a classic addictive challenge. Vigilance is victory here. Stay very aware of your body's needs. Know true hunger versus the False Hunger of the False Fix. That hunger check is a lifesaver. Practice it every day!

Many people who work out upon arising in the morning eat about 100 calories worth of a snack beforehand, as they are usually hungry. But if you're not hungry when you wake up in the morning, you may have eaten too late or too much the night before.

In the vulnerable Detox stage, many of my patients find it easier to follow a step-by-step eating plan, full of structure and predictability. Other patients prefer to get a list of foods and customize it themselves. Both approaches are great—as long as they work for you. I want eating itself to be a Healthy Fix for you—a conscious, deliberate, mindful Healthy Fix, one that makes you proud, energetic, and hopeful. You will no longer be tormented and scared or hide from your food—it's time to fix all of that.

The number-one goal of this chapter is to provide you with the tools to create and maintain a lifestyle that puts you on the path to a healthier relationship with food. As you read in Chapter 5, I am a big believer in the power of preparing your own foods—but I'm not here to turn you into a chef. Far from it. As Julia Child once said, "You don't have to cook fancy or complicated masterpieces—just good food from fresh ingredients."

I want to show you that simple preparations can help you redefine food. Holding it, working with it, and appreciating its nourishment are all part of the healing process. As long as you're making the switch from False Fixes to Healthy Fixes, as long as you're more physically active, meditating, journaling, and staying centered, you'll be able to rein in overeating. You'll practice this from the moment you start Detox through the rest of your life.

One of the reasons people still pop diet suppressant pills is because the pills take away not only their appetite but also any interest in food and therefore any need to make choices. Many of my patients are so food phobic that they would rather endure days and weeks of slurping shakes for every meal rather than have to think about food. Sadly, both the shakes and pills are fraught with side effects, yield only short-term results, and then trigger a major rebound of weight gain. You cannot solve your overeating by running away from food. Let's stand together and confront this food-phobia demon in your own kitchen.

Struggling with False Fixes of processed, faux food, you've probably been disconnected from real foods—foods that grew from the earth, foods that don't have a USDA label that reads like you're

bloating, and bowel changes. To minimize discomfort, you must adhere to the template of eating frequent meals and snacks. Drink plenty (8 to 12 cups) of fluids (water, sparkling water, and unsweetened seltzer) throughout the day, and more when you exercise. Keep in mind, these symptoms will decrease as your body adjusts to the amount of fiber ingested.

If discomfort persists, then try unsweetened herbal teas such as ginger, mint, and chamomile. You can also prevent gas and bloating by taking a product like Beano before you eat. This product assists in breaking down raffinose (the indigestible carbohydrate found in fruits, vegetables, legumes, and whole grains) that can cause gas and bloating.

Once you're done with Detox, you'll have the confidence to take on a few more sophisticated dishes, so Stage 2 meals (starting on page 234) will give you a bit of variety and challenge. The foods in Stage 2 still use many dopamine-boosting nutrients, but you'll also expand into more nutrients that support total brain health—such as increased levels of omega-3 fatty acids—to give your neurogenesis some additional raw material to work with.

Once you hit Stage 3, your skills will be sharpened to the point where you will be ready for some seriously mind-blowing recipes. These meals center on methyl donor foods that support positive epigenetic changes, all livened up with spices selected for their exciting taste as well as the biochemical changes they stimulate in the body to help lengthen your life!

With mix-and-match meals, the Hunger Fix eating plan is flexible enough to accommodate unique food preferences, challenging schedules, demanding families, or portions for one, and even for those who really don't like to cook. The foods will delight the senses in a healthy way and open your eyes to how delicious and satisfying whole, healthy, nonaddictive food can be.

The Hunger Fix plan knows that the way to freedom is lined with pleasure—so pull up a chair and dig in!

(continued on page 223)

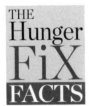

Rounding Up the Raw Materials

You're going to start Stage 1 by stocking your kitchen with healthy, nutrient-dense ingredients. You'll need the ingredients below to make the recipes—and if you build your pantry around these items, you can't go wrong.

Oils and Vinegars

Most fats that are liquid at room temperature (oils) are primarily composed of healthier unsaturated fats. The Hunger Fix recipes are low in saturated fat because they use oils rather than butter. Oils are susceptible to oxidation and should be stored in a cool, dark place (*not* over the stove). Oils with higher smoke points are appropriate for cooking; oils with lower smoke points are better used in dressings or for drizzling. Vinegars can provide flavor and tang to dressings and dishes. Zesty!

- Cooking oils: olive, canola, peanut, and sesame
- Drizzling oils: extra-virgin olive oil, nut oils; cold pressed or infused
- Vinegars: balsamic, rice wine, sherry, champagne, distilled, and cider

Nuts and Seeds

Nuts and seeds are powerhouse sources of vitamins, minerals, protein, fiber, and healthy fats—and may extend your life by 3 years.[2] When available, they should be purchased raw or roasted without salt. Store them in the freezer if you buy them in bulk. You can roast nuts easily at home. Seeds are also good additions to salads, snack mixes, muffins, or smoothies. Flaxseeds and chia seeds are sources of healthy omega-3 fatty acids. Some seeds, such as flaxseeds, need to be ground to increase the bioavailability of the nutrients in the seeds.

- Nuts: almonds, peanuts, walnuts, hazelnuts, pecans, cashews, and Brazil nuts
- Seeds: chia, sunflower, pumpkin, and flaxseeds

Grains and Cereals

Buy only whole, intact grains or flours made from 100 percent whole grain. While some vitamins and minerals are added back as part of the enrichment process, whole, intact grains have more vitamins, minerals, protein, and fiber than their refined counterparts. Popcorn can be popped with no oil in an air popper and topped with a small amount of healthy oil and a wide variety of flavors and spices (see page 222). Wheat germ and oat bran add nutritious crunch to cereal, yogurt, and muffins.

- Whole, intact grains: stone-ground oats, wheat berries, barley, brown rice, quinoa, bulgur, and popcorn kernels
- Wheat germ and oat bran

While intact grains are always best, processed grain products such as breads, pastas, and crackers are included less frequently in the meal plans. Look for products that say "100%" and read ingredient labels to see if the flours or grains used in the product are whole.

- 100 percent whole wheat or white whole wheat flour (available from King Arthur or Bob's Red Mill), whole wheat pasta, 100 percent whole grain breads, 100 percent whole grain cereals with no added sugar, whole wheat bread crumbs

Cooking Stocks

Cooking stocks give foods greater depth of flavor. Commercial stocks available in the grocery store can be high in sodium—look for low-sodium varieties. Save money by using the basic stock recipes made from cooking scraps! (See the Hunger Fix Food Fact "Making Your Own Stock" on page 240.) Making fresh stock allows you to control the sodium and added ingredients. Make it in bulk and freeze it for up to 3 months.

- Stock: chicken, seafood, beef, and vegetable

Sweeteners

Sugars and sweeteners are used sparingly in the recipes in this chapter. Agave syrup has a more intense sweetness and therefore you can use less to achieve the same level of sweetness.

- Honey, brown sugar, granulated sugar, and agave syrup

Beans, Legumes, and Nut Butters

Beans and legumes are among the least expensive and most nutrient-dense foods available. Buy low- or no-sodium cans or drain and rinse the beans to remove excess salt. Dried beans are even more inexpensive and with a little forethought, just as easy to prepare. (See the Hunger Fix Food Fact "Cooking Dried Legumes" on page 238.)

- Canned or dried: kidney beans, chickpeas, pinto beans, black beans, white beans, split peas, lentils, and black-eyed peas
  Note: Heritage or heirloom beans can be found in gourmet groceries or online.

Used in the appropriate portions, nut butters provide healthy fats and protein with little additional carbohydrates. Look for brands without partially hydrogenated fats added. The oil in an all-natural nut butter separates on top and needs to be stirred prior to refrigeration.

- Peanut, almond, and cashew

(continued)

The Hunger Fix Facts—*Continued*

Dairy and Plant Milks

Dairy products provide potassium, vitamins A and D, and protein—but also saturated fat. Plant milks also contain protein but without the saturated fat and are fortified with many of the vitamins found in milk. Milks should be unflavored unless specified in the recipe. Fat-free or low-fat dairy is best. Greek yogurt has more protein than regular plain yogurt—mix it with fruit and skip the corn-syrup-laden commercially sweetened kinds.

- Fat-free Greek yogurt, low-fat cottage cheese, low-fat cheese, and 1% or fat-free milk

- Soy and almond milk

Animal Proteins

Animal proteins are a source of important amino acids like tyrosine, the building block of dopamine. Protein helps us feel full and satisfied and keeps blood sugar on an even keel, so we don't go into withdrawal. If you're new to cooking, try to get past any fear of bone-in meats—these cost-effective cuts provide scraps for stock, and roasting with the bone in keeps meat juicy. Look for 100 percent pasture-raised meats, especially beef, as they have more omega-3s and other healthy fats than their grain-finished counterparts. Visit your local farmers' market and ask the farmer how the animals are raised. This chapter provides basic recipes for preparing various cuts of chicken, turkey, pork, lean beef, and fish. The chicken, turkey, and pork can be prepared in larger quantities and then used over the week in salads or soups as directed in the recipes.

Eggs have gotten a bad rap because they are high in dietary cholesterol. However, they are an excellent source of nutrients, including protein and omega-3 fats. If possible, look for pastured eggs or purchase eggs from local farmers at a farmers' market where you can ask the farmer how the chickens are kept. Eggs from pasture-raised chickens are naturally higher in omega-3 fatty acids and healthier fats.

Another way to increase the protein in a meal is with protein powder. Found in many grocery stores, health food stores, or online, protein powders can be added to soups, stews, yogurt, smoothies, and cooked cereals.

- Poultry: whole chicken, legs, breast, and ground
- Fish: fresh fish, canned tuna, salmon, and sardines
- Lean beef: loin
- Pork: loin, tenderloin, and chop
- Shellfish: shrimp
- Eggs
- Protein powder: egg, whey, and soy

Produce

Fruits and vegetables are king! Low in calories, high in fiber, packed with vitamins, minerals, and phytochemicals, produce is the foundation of the Hunger Fix eating plan. All produce tastes best in season, so explore your local farmers' market for deliciously timed fare. (A ripe peach in July? Perfection!)

Keep lemons, garlic, onions, celery, and carrots on hand all the time—these are staples in your well-equipped kitchen. Fruits, especially berries, are best eaten in season but can be purchased in bulk and frozen (freeze each in a single layer on a baking sheet and then store in freezer bags). Frozen edamame and peas are also easy sources of protein to toss into many recipes. Dried fruits such as prunes, cherries, raisins, apple rings, apricots, and figs can make healthy snacks—but their sweetness can lead to binges. Beware! Look for options with no added sugar or sulfites.

Here's some information on storing produce, as it's a major issue when you're transitioning to fresh foods for the first time. Check this chart and you won't go wrong.

Ripen on Counter, Then Refrigerate	Store in Refrigerator Crisper Drawer, in Unsealed Plastic Bag/Container		Store out of Direct Sunlight in Cool, Dark Place
• Apricots	• Asparagus**	• Green beans	• Garlic
• Avocados	• Beets	• Herbs**	• Jicama
• Apples	• Blueberries	• Kale	• Onions
• Bananas*	• Broccoli	• Leeks	• Potatoes
• Grapefruit	• Brussels sprouts	• Lettuce	• Shallots
• Guava	• Cabbage	• Mushrooms***	• Sweet potatoes
• Kiwifruit	• Carrots	• Okra***	• Tomatoes
• Lemons	• Cauliflower	• Peas	• Winter squash
• Limes	• Celery	• Peppers	• Yuca
• Oranges	• Chard	• Radishes	
• Papaya	• Cherries	• Raspberries	*Skin may brown in the refrigerator, but the fruit will remain firm.
• Peaches	• Collard greens	• Scallions	
• Pears	• Corn	• Spinach	**Wrap ends in a damp paper towel or place in a jar of water.
• Pineapple	• Cucumbers	• Strawberries	
• Plums	• Eggplant	• Summer squash	***Store in a paper bag.[3]
	• Figs	• Rutabagas	
	• Ginger	• Turnips	
	• Grapes	• Zucchini	

(continued)

Herbs and Condiments

Spices and fresh herbs add calorie-free flavor that delight your reward center—and phytochemicals that delight the rest of your body! Dried, ground spices and herbs should be kept away from heat sources (such as next to the stove) and replaced annually. Whole spices will keep their flavors for much longer, so if you can, purchase whole spices in bulk and grind them in a spice grinder (or a coffee grinder dedicated to spices). Fresh herbs should be stored in water or in a slightly damp towel in the refrigerator. These all add a delicious zing to the Hunger Fix recipes.

- Spices: cayenne, chili powder, cumin, cinnamon, curry, smoked paprika, dry mustard, nutmeg, red pepper flakes, ginger, turmeric, celery seed, and cloves

- Herbs: dill, parsley, cilantro, basil, oregano, chives, and scallions

- Condiments: mustard (yellow and Dijon), hot sauce, chipotle hot sauce, soy sauce, Worcestershire sauce, and mayonnaise

Stage 1

DETOX BREAKFASTS

The first 2 to 4 weeks are all about kicking those False Fixes—easily and without stress. You'll notice that none of these breakfasts require you to prepare a recipe—they're simply grab-and-go. No excuses to skip! A hearty breakfast with protein, healthy fat, and soluble fiber will set you up for energy throughout the morning, so you can resist the bagel shop or pastry cart and keep going until lunch.

- 1–1½ cups fat-free Greek yogurt, 1 ounce walnuts, 1 medium banana
- 2 tablespoons peanut butter on 2 Wasa crackers, smoothie made with 8 ounces milk, 2 tablespoons protein powder, ½ banana
- 1 package oatmeal with 2 tablespoons protein powder, 1 tablespoon walnuts, 1 cup fruit salad
- 2 hard-cooked eggs, 1–1½ cups fresh fruit salad, 1 packet low-sugar oatmeal
- 2 scrambled eggs, 1 package oatmeal, and 1–1½ cups fruit salad
- 1–1½ cups fat-free Greek yogurt, 1 ounce almonds, 1 tablespoon chia seeds, 1 cup strawberries
- 1–1½ cups fat-free cottage cheese, 1 tablespoon shredded coconut, 1½ cups pineapple, ½ cup high-fiber cereal
- 2 hard-cooked eggs, 1 cup high-fiber cereal, 8 ounces milk, 1 cup blueberries
- 2 tablespoons almond butter on 4 Wasa crackers, 1 cup fat-free cottage cheese, 1 peach
- 1–1½ cups fat-free cottage cheese, 2 tablespoons chia seeds, 1–1½ cups cantaloupe
- 2 hard-cooked eggs, 1 apple, 1 slice whole wheat toast with 1 tablespoon peanut butter

- 3-egg omelet with 1 tablespoon each of ham, bell pepper, and onion and 1 slice of whole wheat toast

- 1 tablespoon peanut butter on 1 banana rolled in 1 tablespoon wheat germ in 1–1½ cups Greek yogurt

- 1–1½ cups fat-free cottage cheese, 2 tablespoons almonds, 1–1½ cups grapes

- 1–1½ cups fat-free Greek yogurt, 1 ounce pecans, 1 tablespoon flax meal, 1 cup sliced peaches

- Smoothie: 2 tablespoons peanut butter, ½ banana, 12 ounces milk, 2 tablespoons protein powder, 1 tablespoon flax meal

- 2 hard-cooked eggs, smoothie (½ cup blueberries, ½ cup strawberries, 1 tablespoon protein powder, 8 ounces milk)

- 1–1½ cups fat-free cottage cheese, 2 tablespoons walnuts, 1–1½ cups raspberries

- 3–egg white omelet with ½ cup mushrooms and 2 tablespoons shredded cheese over 1 slice whole wheat toast, 1 cup grapes

- 2 hard-cooked eggs, 1 banana rolled in 1 tablespoon peanut butter and 1 tablespoon wheat germ

- 1–1½ cups fat-free Greek yogurt, 1 ounce pecans, 1 tablespoon wheat germ, 1 cup blueberries

- 1 scrambled egg on whole wheat English muffin, 1 slice ham, 1–1½ cups melon

- 2 hard-cooked eggs, 1 cup fruit salad, 1 cup Greek yogurt

- 1–1½ cups fat-free cottage cheese, 2 tablespoons flax meal, 1 cup mango

- 3 scrambled egg whites on 1 slice whole wheat toast, 1 slice Swiss cheese, 1 orange

- 2 tablespoons almond butter on 1 whole wheat English muffin, 1 apple, 2 scrambled egg whites

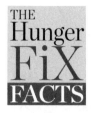

The Macronutrient Mix

The Hunger Fix eating plan works with an average 20 to 30 percent of calories from protein, 25 to 35 percent from fat, and 30 to 35 percent from carbohydrate. The meal plan is packed with foods that build dopamine and positively alter gene expression to aid in satiety, reduce cravings, and keep you on the path to success. But all that is factored in automatically—all you have to do is eat and enjoy.

Proteins provide amino acids, such as tyrosine and phenylalanine, to protect your dopamine supply. Protein triggers satiety, a critical part of satisfying meals and snacks. To get your 20 to 30 percent protein, you'll focus on lean sources such as beans, fish, poultry, and eggs, packed with the nutrient choline, the building block of other helpful neurotransmitters, such as acetylcholine and serotonin.

Fat may have more calories per gram than protein or carbohydrates, but eating fat at breakfast may keep your fat metabolism stoked during the day. Your brain is composed of fat, so healthy omega-3 fats are essential for health—you can get them only from your diet. The Hunger Fix plan provides 25 to 35 percent of calories from fat, mostly from beneficial oils and proteins.

Carbohydrates are in grains, dairy, fruit (and juice), low-starch vegetables, and any sugar—and many processed foods. A clear culprit in most food False Fixes, sugars and refined grains are a big no-no; even whole grains can trigger addictions for some. Aim to get your 35 to 45 percent of carbs from fruit, veggies, and low-fat dairy, and keep all grains, pastas, breads, and potatoes to a minimum.

Note: To help address common lingering nutrient deficiencies, please consider taking a high quality multivitamin, omega 3 supplements, vitamin D, calcium fortified with D, and probiotics. Please talk with your doctor about the correct dosages for these supplements to suit your own unique health situation.

- 1–1½ cups fat-free Greek yogurt, 1 ounce almonds, 1 tablespoon chia seeds, 1 cup blackberries
- 2 sunny-side-up eggs over 1 slice whole wheat toast, 1 cup pineapple

Stage 1

DETOX LUNCHES

Lunch is another quick meal often consumed away from home: at your desk, in the car, or on the go. Too many high-calorie foods can inhibit your afternoon performance, leaving you feeling sluggish all afternoon. Most people plan a snack for midafternoon, so lunch should just tide you over until then. The strategy for lunch includes a variety of delicious soups and salads that contain those key lean proteins, soluble fiber, and healthy fats. We have included recipes, but not everyone will have or make the time to prepare them. Many acceptable soups and salads can be found at grocery stores, delis, diners, salad bars, corporate cafeterias, and so on. The Hunger Fix recipes will provide a guide of what ingredients and types of soups and salads to look for if you don't have the time for preparation at home.

- 1 grilled chicken breast, $\frac{1}{2}$ avocado, $\frac{1}{2}$ cup black beans
- 1–1$\frac{1}{2}$ cups Chicken Salad (page 258), made with Greek yogurt, over 2 cups romaine, $\frac{1}{2}$ toasted whole wheat pita
- 4–6 ounces grilled salmon, 1–1$\frac{1}{2}$ cups steamed cauliflower, $\frac{1}{2}$ cup brown rice
- 4–6 ounces rotisserie chicken breast, 1–1$\frac{1}{2}$ cups steamed mixed vegetables, $\frac{1}{2}$–$\frac{1}{3}$ cup kidney beans
- 4–6 ounces chicken breast with $\frac{1}{2}$–$\frac{3}{4}$ cup black beans and 1 cup chopped tomato, 1 tablespoon crumbled feta, 1 teaspoon olive oil, and 2 tablespoons red wine vinegar
- 3–4 slices lean roast beef, each rolled up with 1 ounce roasted red peppers and a touch of mustard; 1 cup Three Bean Salad (page 259); 2 whole grain sesame thins
- 2 cups spinach salad with 2 teaspoons olive oil and 1 tablespoon balsamic vinegar, 4–6 ounces Crispy Tofu (page 259), a $\frac{1}{2}$ cup bulgur

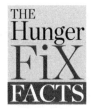

Fixate on Fiber

While fiber is one of the top weight-loss aids on earth, and the USDA recommends 25 to 35 grams of fiber per day, the typical American diet includes merely 10 grams—so we have some work to do! As you follow the Hunger Fix eating plan, be sure that you're drinking plenty of water (8 to 12 cups a day) to help your system adjust to all the fiber you'll get from whole foods. While I recommend caution with grains, when you do eat them, always choose whole, intact grains (brown rice, whole barley, quinoa, faro, spelt) instead of bread, pasta, or cereal. If you must eat the latter, look for whole grains (not whole grain *flour*) in the ingredients.

Soluble fiber attracts water in our digestive system and forms a gel, making us feel full and slowing down digestion. Soluble fiber is also beneficial in that it can help lower cholesterol and is associated with a low glycemic index that has a positive effect on insulin sensitivity (good news for all of us—especially those with high blood sugar). While soluble fiber can be tricky to find, it's worth it—studies have found that if you increase your soluble fiber by 10 grams per day (the amount in two servings of beans, an apple, and a pear), you could reduce your LDL by 5 percent[4] and your toxic belly fat by 3.7 percent.

Sources include: oats, dried beans and legumes (lentils, black/white/pinto/kidney/garbanzo beans/peas), broccoli (and other crucifers), brown rice, popcorn, chia seeds, citrus, apricots, nuts, barley, flaxseeds, apples, pears, oranges, strawberries, blueberries, cucumbers, celery, carrots, and psyllium.

Insoluble fiber is great for digestion—it does not dissolve in water and so speeds up the passage of food and waste through the digestive tract, like a broom sweeping out our insides. Insoluble fiber is more common than soluble; it's found in almost every plant food.

Sources include: wheat bran, corn bran, brown rice, leafy greens, grapes, raisins, zucchini, cruciferous vegetables (broccoli, cauliflower, and cabbage), nuts, seeds, and the skins of fruits and root vegetables.

- Salad bar: 1 cup greens, 1–1½ cups raw veggies (peppers, cucumbers, tomatoes, carrots, mushrooms), ¼ cup beans (black, kidney, chickpeas), 1 cup protein (chicken, egg, cottage cheese, ham, tofu), 1 tablespoon each of nuts and dried fruit; drizzle of olive oil (not over 2 teaspoons) and 1 tablespoon vinegar (balsamic, red, or white)

- Open-faced turkey sandwich: 4 ounces warmed turkey breast over 1 slice toasted whole grain bread, 1 slice melted Swiss, 8–12 ounces Vegetable Soup (page 260)

- 1–1½ cups Egg Salad with Greek Yogurt (page 258) over 2 cups romaine, 4 Wasa crackers

- 10–16 ounces Minestrone Soup (page 261), 4 whole grain crackers, 1–1½ cups spinach salad

- 10–16 ounces Chicken Vegetable Soup (page 262), ½ cup wild rice blend

- 4–6 ounces shrimp, ½ cup brown rice, 1–1½ cups steamed mixed vegetables

- 4–6 ounces grilled salmon, ½ cup barley, 1–1½ cups steamed asparagus

- 4–6 ounces grilled chicken breast, 8–12 ounces Vegetable Soup (page 260), 4 whole grain crackers

- 4 ounces turkey breast, 1 slice Swiss cheese, 2 cups garden salad and 2 teaspoons olive oil and 1 tablespoon vinegar, 2 Wasa crackers

- Open-faced roast beef sandwich (3–4 slices lean roast beef and ½ teaspoon mustard on 1 slice rye bread), 2 cups garden salad with 2 teaspoons olive oil and 1 tablespoon red wine vinegar

- 4–6 ounces baked cod, 1–1½ cups steamed green beans, 1 cup roasted potatoes

- 4–6 ounces roast pork, 1½ cups steamed broccoli, ½ cup brown rice

- 4–6 ounces canned salmon, 1 cup edamame, 1–1½ cups carrot sticks

- 4–6 ounces tilapia, 2–3 cups garden salad with 2 teaspoons olive oil and 1 tablespoon vinegar, ½ cup brown rice

- Grilled chicken garden salad: 4–6 ounces grilled chicken over 2–3 cups garden salad with lettuce, tomatoes, cucumber, carrots,

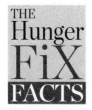

Easy Tweaks for Vegetarians

While some of the meals included in the plans are vegetarian, most can be adjusted to accommodate a vegetarian diet. In the lunch soups, vegetable stock can be substituted for the chicken, meat, or fish stocks used in the recipes. Protein powder and plant-based proteins such as tofu, textured vegetable protein, seitan, or tempeh can be used in place of the poultry, fish, or meat in the meal. Protein powders can be added to smoothies in the morning to provide additional protein. The recipe for Crispy Tofu (page 259) is one way to prepare firm tofu so that it can be used in a variety of meals. Silken tofu can be pureed into soups for added protein.

and peppers, 2 teaspoons olive oil, and 1 tablespoon vinegar; 2 Wasa crackers

- 4–6 ounces grilled salmon, 1½ cups mixed steamed vegetables, ½ cup brown rice

- Open-faced tuna melt: 1–1½ cups Tuna Salad with Greek Yogurt (page 258), 1 slice toasted whole wheat bread with 1 slice Swiss cheese, garden salad

- 1–1½ cups Tuna Salad with Greek Yogurt (page 258) over 2 cups romaine, 4 Wasa crackers

- 4–6 ounces grilled chicken, ½–¾ cup chickpeas, 1–2 cups fresh vegetables (from salad bar)

- 4–6 ounces tilapia, two 6-inch whole wheat or corn tortillas, ½ cup tomatoes, 1 cup lettuce, ½ avocado, ¼ cup salsa

- 4–6 ounces grilled sirloin, 1–1½ cups steamed broccoli, ½ cup brown rice

Stage 1

DINNERS

The Hunger Fix dinners are no-stress moments to relax and enjoy. While preparing your meal, your senses will be inundated with the aroma, colors, and textures of the dish. Many people find that once it comes time to actually sit down and eat, this sensory infusion helps them eat less. Ideally, preparing dinner will become a joyous Healthy Fix in and of itself. Some prep and cook times may be longer, but I've tried to keep the active prep time to a minimum for most recipes in this book. And remember: Leftovers can quickly be turned into tomorrow's lunch.

Cooking your own food gives you complete control of what ingredients you choose—no guessing how much oil, salt, or sugar is being added to a dish. But when you do have to catch a meal on the go, look for menu items that mimic these meal plans.

You may notice that this eating plan avoids grains at night. I find these can trigger False Fix carb cravings and set up a pattern of late-night snacking that many folks find hard to break. Traditionally, dinner is our biggest meal of the day, but it's actually best to taper down your food intake at night to avoid acid reflux and set yourself up for a better night of sleep. If you have an early dinner, you can have a snack 2 hours before bed—but if dinner is past 7:00 p.m., it should be your last eating occasion. As soon as possible thereafter, brush your teeth, and consider taking a shower and putting on your PJs right away—this will signal to your brain that eating time is over and rest time has begun.

- 4–6 ounces baked salmon, 1–1½ cups steamed brussels sprouts
- 4–6 ounces roasted chicken breast, 1–1½ cups steamed cauliflower
- 4–6 ounces turkey breast, 1–1½ cups steamed mixed vegetables (page 233)

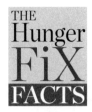

Kit Out Your Kitchen

Below is a list of kitchen tools to start your cooking adventures off right! If you don't have all of these tools to start, never fear—consider acquiring one tool a week (or a month) as a reward for learning new skills! While most widely available tools do the job, I have recommended some brands I like in my own kitchen. For fun once you hit Stage 3, visit a restaurant supply store—you'll be amazed how much more you can know about kitchen tools and what they can do!

- Cutting board
- Handheld stick blender with mini-food processor and whip (Cuisinart Smart Stick)
- High-quality utility knife (santoku style—Wüsthof [very pricey!] and J.A. Henckels [also expensive, but less so])
- Large ovenproof sauté pan with lid
- Measuring cups up to 1 quart
- Measuring spoons
- Mixing bowls (various sizes)
- Mortar and pestle
- Nonstick skillet
- Ovenproof Dutch oven
- Snap glassware containers
- Steaming basket
- Stockpot
- Tongs
- Vegetable peeler (Kuhn Rikon)
- Heavy-duty blender (Vita-Prep)
- Zester

- 4–6 ounces grilled tilapia, 1–1½ cups steamed asparagus
- 6–8 ounces Crispy Tofu (page 259), 1–1½ cups steamed mixed vegetables (page 233)

- 4–6 ounces baked turkey breast, 1–1½ cups roasted beets
- 4–6 ounces sliced sirloin, 1–1½ cups steamed carrots and sugar snap peas
- 4–6 ounces grilled salmon, 1–1½ cups Roasted Butternut Squash (page 283)
- 4–6 ounces pork loin, 1–1½ cups Roasted Butternut Squash (page 283)
- 4–6 ounces baked chicken legs, 1–1½ cups steamed green beans
- 4–6 ounces shrimp, 1–1½ cups steamed Asian vegetables
- 4–6 ounces baked salmon, 1–1½ cups steamed broccoli
- 4 to 6 grilled chicken breast, 1–1½ cups steamed summer squash
- 4–6 ounces pork tenderloin, 1–1½ cups steamed brussels sprouts
- 4–6 ounces pork chop, 1–1½ cups sautéed spinach (see opposite)
- 4–6 ounces sirloin slices, 1–1½ cups sautéed spinach (see opposite)
- 4–6 ounces sautéed shrimp, 1–1½ cups broccoli
- 4–6 ounces grilled tuna steak, 2–3 cups Greek Salad (page 284) with 1 tablespoon feta cheese, 2 teaspoons olive oil, and 1 tablespoon red wine vinegar
- 6–8 ounces Crispy Tofu (page 259), 1–1½ cups steamed broccoli and mushrooms
- 4–6 ounces baked chicken legs, 1–1½ cups steamed carrots
- 4–6 ounces grilled salmon, 1–1½ cups raw vegetable salad (cucumbers, tomatoes, peppers) with 1 teaspoon olive oil and 2 teaspoons vinegar
- 4–6 ounces chicken breast, 1–1½ cups steamed Asian vegetables
- 4–6 ounces turkey breast, 1 small baked sweet potato
- 4–6 ounces baked flounder; 1–1½ cups stewed tomatoes, peppers, and onion
- 4–6 ounces baked chicken breast, 1 cup Wilted Swiss Chard (page 284) and garlic, ¼ cup black beans

unces Herbed Mustard Salmon (page 285), 1–1½ cups
d brussels sprouts (page 233)

unces tilapia prepared with Hot and Spicy Marinade (page
1–1½ cups Broccoli with Garlic and Ginger (page 286)

unces pork loin prepared with Red Wine Marinade (page
1–1½ cups Roasted Butternut Squash (page 283)

ups Shrimp Stir-Fry (page 287)

ounces Turkey Meat Loaf (page 288), 1–1½ cups Roasted
iflower (page 289)

ounces whole roasted chicken (see opposite), 1–1½ cups
n Beans with Roasted Garlic and Lemon (page 290)

ounces marinated sirloin steak, 1–1½ cups sautéed spinach

Basic Tips for Cooking Chicken

Cooking chicken breast on the bone with the skin
results in a moister, more flavorful chicken breast. Preheat
the oven to 375°F. Place the breasts in a baking dish or
pan, skin side up. Season with ¼ teaspoon each of salt
and pepper. For small breasts, bake for 40 minutes. For
large breasts, bake for 55 minutes. Let the chicken rest 5
es before serving. Removing the skin after cooking decreases
s, fat, and saturated fat.

neless, skinless chicken breast can be more expensive but a bit
to get past picky eaters. Preheat the oven to 375°F. Coat a 10-inch
roof skillet with cooking spray. Season each side of the breast with
spoon each of salt and pepper. In the skillet on the stove, over
m heat, sear one side of the breasts for 3 minutes. Flip the breasts,
place the skillet in the oven for 15 to 20 minutes, depending upon the
ess of the breast. Let the chicken rest 5 minutes before serving.

neless, skinless chicken legs have a more intense flavor. Preheat
ven to 350°F. Coat a baking dish or pan with cooking spray. Place the
en legs in one layer, leaving about ½ inch in between pieces. Season
¼ teaspoon each of salt and pepper. Cover with foil. Bake for 35 to 40
tes. Keep the chicken covered until serving to prevent drying out.

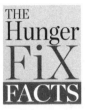

Cooking Vegetables

Fresh, seasonal vegetables are standard for most of the
Hunger Fix recipes. However, some vegetables are not
always in season or easy to find. You can substitute frozen
veggies when needed, especially in soups. Remember
that many frozen vegetables are already cooked so they
should be added toward the end of cooking. Frozen peas
and spinach are especially useful and versatile. Look for plain vegetables—
they should be the sole ingredient in the package, without any added salt
or sauces. Here are some veggie-cooking methods you'll use throughout
the Hunger Fix plan.

Steaming just requires an inexpensive steaming basket (available at most
grocery stores) that fits inside a variety of pots. Pour a few inches of water in
the pan, turn the stove heat up to high, and pile the vegetables in the basket.
Steam until the veggies are tender but firm—mushy veggies don't always
have quite the reward factor. Steaming works for almost any vegetable, but
cook times vary, so test for desired doneness by poking veggies with a knife
or carefully taste testing until you're satisfied with the consistency.

Sautéing sounds exotic, but it just means cooking in a pan or wok with
a small amount of oil (a few teaspoons) or cooking spray over medium to
medium-high heat. Again, different vegetables require different cook
times. Sautéing is great for vegetables that cook quickly, such as
mushrooms, summer squash, and greens; it also builds savory flavors with
the browning that occurs, especially if you use garlic, onions, and other
ingredients.

Roasting is a dry cooking method done in the oven in a baking dish or
sheet pan. Roasting concentrates flavors and—bonus!—the oven does the
work while you do other things! Root vegetables, broccoli, cauliflower,
brussels sprouts, and carrots all taste great roasted. Just toss them with a
small amount of oil or coat them with cooking spray and some salt, pepper,
and other spices before roasting. (*Tip:* Line the pan with foil for easy
cleanup.)

- 4–6 ounces pork tenderloin, 1–1½ cups steamed sugar snap peas
- 4–6 ounces sliced chicken breast, 2 cups mixed greens with
  2 teaspoons olive oil and ½ cup chickpeas
- 4–6 ounces grilled salmon, 1–1½ cups roasted asparagus, 1 small
  baked potato

Stage 2

Stage 2 is all about practice, practice, practice. You have the option of sticking with the simple Stage 1 meals or expanding your meal and snack choices in this stage. Do whatever feels safe and comfortable for you. The breakfast options are exactly the same in Stage 2 and Stage 3, so refer to page 223 for those options. For Stages 2 and 3, I'll give you a week of menus each, so you can get a hang of what the meals look like. (Check out my Web site at www.drpeeke.com for more Stages 2 and 3 meals as well as a couple of interesting breakfast options.) As you become comfortable with the recipes in Phases 2 and 3, you'll find they can easily be tweaked and customized to your satisfaction. Make sure to rotate fish, poultry, meat, and vegetarian meal options so your body gets a variety of nutrients.

Stage 2

LUNCHES

- 10–16 ounces Turkey Chili (page 264), 1 cup fresh berries

- 10–16 ounces Smoky Tomato Bean Soup (page 263), 1–1½ cups Crispy Tofu Carrot Salad (page 265)

- 10–16 ounces Rhode Island Chowder (page 266), 1–1½ cups Three Bean Salad (page 259)

- Open-faced turkey sandwich: 4 ounces warmed turkey breast and 1 slice melted Swiss cheese over 1 slice toasted whole grain bread; with 8–12 ounces Minestrone Soup (page 261)

- 10–16 ounces Lentil Soup (page 267), 1–1½ cups Roasted Beets (page 268)

- 10–16 ounces Broccoli Cheddar Soup with Chicken (page 269), 1–1½ cups Chickpea Salad (page 270)

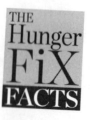

Cooking Gr[...]

Whole grains are m[...]
top. Quinoa, barley, a[...]
to cooking—be sure [...]
any small stones or d[...]
whole grains is to use[...]
1 cup of grain—but be[...]
whenever they're available. With most [...]
to the pot and then cover with the lid[...]
couscous, you bring the water to a boil [...]

For intact grains, bring the pot of grai[...]
high heat and then reduce the heat to [...]
grain, the cooking time can be as quick [...]
long as 30 to 45 minutes (brown rice ar[...]
require less time and heat to cook—once [...]
covered and removed from the heat.

Cooked grains should be tender but no[...]
enough by the end of the cooking time, [...]
stock and continue cooking. Be sure the p[...]
too long without any liquid in the bottom [...]
bottom of pot!

To build flavor in a grain dish, use a st[...]
fragrant spices (such as nutmeg, cinnam[...]
chopped vegetables (such as onions, garlic,[...]
in the pot with a small amount of oil prior to [...]

- 10–16 ounces Hearty Southwestern Chi[...]
  1–1½ cups Sweet and Spicy Slaw (page [...]

- 4–6 o[...]
  roaste[...]

- 4–6 o[...]
  255),[...]

- 4–6 o[...]
  256),[...]

- 2–3 o[...]

- 4–6 [...]
  Cau[...]

- 4–6 [...]
  Gre[...]

- 4–6 [...]

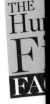

minut[...]
calorie[...]
  Bo[...]
easie[...]
ovenp[...]
¼ tea[...]
medi[...]
then [...]
thick[...]
  Bo[...]
the o[...]
chick[...]
with [...]
minu[...]

Stage 3

In Phase 3, we will build on what we learned in Phase 2, with a few new techniques and ingredients. Now that your 80 percent weight-loss goal has been achieved, you can further expand your safe foods. In the best of all worlds, you're still cooking your meals when you can so that ingredients and portions are carefully monitored.

Many recovering food addicts feel "safe" only when they keep things quite simple, even for many years after dropping significant weight. Others are a bit more adventuresome but still have food terrors and fear becoming fat again should a food trigger their addiction. Therefore, the food plans and recipes for this stage span the spectrum from very simple Stage 1 plans (see page 223) to more expansive Stage 2 offerings (see page 234). Note that throughout the Hunger Fix eating plan, you can always scoot back to Stage 1: Detox meals if you find yourself getting a little out of control. In Stage 3 meals, we'll expand into a more intermediate cooking level experience, adding a bit higher level to the food plans and recipes, since your body (and mind) is now ready to explore more interesting food selections and preparations.

Stage 3

LUNCHES

- 10–16 ounces Gazpacho (page 273), 1–1½ cups Waldorf Salad (page 274) with 4–6 ounces chicken breast

- 10–16 ounces Mushroom Soup (page 275), 1–1½ cups Greek Salad (page 284)

- Swordfish Kebabs (page 276) over 1–1½ cups Cucumber and Lentil Salad (page 277)

- 10–16 ounces Chicken Escarole Soup (page 278), 1–1½ cups Italian Farro Salad (page 279)

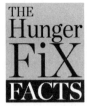

Cooking Dried Legumes

Legumes (beans, peas, lentils) can be cooked in a pot on the stove top. Similar in treatment to grains, beans should be rinsed and picked through to remove debris and shriveled and broken beans. Scout out and remove any floating beans—they're likely hollow or otherwise bunk.

Soaking your beans will shorten your cook times tremendously. Just place them in a full pot of water overnight—no salt, nada. That's it! When you start to cook, discard the soaking water and start again with fresh water.

To cook your beans, cover them with a few inches of water and bring the pot to a boil, then reduce to a simmer. (Toss in a dash of salt, if you like.) As with grains, cooking with stock, a bay leaf, or an herb sachet will add flavor. Cook times will vary bean by bean and will even depend on the freshness of the bean—so keep checking the pot and add water as necessary until the beans are tender. Typical cooking time for soaked beans is 15 to 45 minutes, maybe more for larger beans. More time is required for cooking unsoaked beans—so don't forget to presoak!

- 4–6 ounces Miso Citrus Salmon (page 280) over 1–1½ cups Asian slaw (page 272), 4 whole wheat saltine crackers

- 10–16 ounces Beef Barley Soup (page 281), 1–1½ cups Waldorf Salad (page 274)

- 2–3 cups Asian Shrimp Noodle Salad (page 282)

Stage 3

DINNERS

- 10–16 ounces Cioppino (page 292), 1 ounce Whole Grain Croutons (page 293), 1–2 cups garden salad
- 4–6 ounces Turkey Meatballs (page 294) with sauce, 1–1½ cups sautéed zucchini (page 233)
- 2–3 cups Chicken Stir-Fry (page 287)
- 4–6 ounces Stuffed Flounder (page 295), 1–1½ cups Roasted Asparagus (page 297)
- 2–3 cups Lasagna (page 296)
- 4–6 ounces shrimp prepared with Hot and Spicy Marinade (page 255), 1–1½ cups Broccoli with Garlic and Ginger (page 286)
- 2–3 cups Shepherd's Pie (page 298), 1–1½ cups roasted brussels sprouts (page 233)

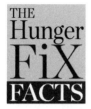

Making Your Own Stock

Cooking with stocks is a very healthy way to add flavor without adding many calories. Store-bought stocks can be expensive and unnecessarily high in sodium, but homemade stock really helps you save money and save the earth, too! Nothing is wasted—you use cooking scraps that would otherwise end up on a landfill, and when prepared with bones, stock will contain more essential nutrients such as calcium, phosphorus, magnesium, sulfur, potassium, chondroitin, keratin, lysine, and other minerals that may be lacking in our diet.

Stocks boast the ultimate "wing it" recipes. There are no fussy measurements—just a couple of tips to follow.

For meat stock, toss leftover roasted bones (with or without meat), some vegetables like onion, carrot, and celery, and a few cups of water into a small pot. You can also add parsley, ginger peels, garlic, and scallions that may be past their prime. No salt necessary! Boil the stock gently for about an hour or so (longer is fine). When it has cooled a bit, strain out the solids with a strainer and/or cheesecloth. Divide the stock into containers that can be stored in the fridge or freezer. That's it! Some tips:

- For a vegetable stock, simply omit the bones.

- Seafood stocks can be made using shrimp or lobster shells in place of bones.

- Leftover bones that have been eaten off of, from your plate, are perfect for stocks. Not gross at all! They're submerged in boiling water so no need to worry about germs.

- Scraps of vegetables are great to use. Toss it all in: carrot ends and peels, celery ends and leaves, onion skins (give great color!) and ends.

- Drippings from roasted proteins and any other leftover scraps can be added as well—the more, the tastier!

Stage 3

SNACKS

You won't feel deprived or hungry on the Hunger Fix eating plan! Make sure you're eating every 3 to 4 hours to head off any blood sugar dips or feelings of deprivation. Here's a list of balanced snacks that will diminish hunger between meals. I have included options that will satisfy all sorts of cravings, including salty, crunchy, and sweet, among others. The most appropriate times for snacking are between breakfast and lunch and between lunch and dinner—avoid late-night snacking as much as humanly possible.

- 2 cups air-popped popcorn with olive oil and salt/pepper, nutritional yeast, lemon oil, and sea salt or with your favorite spice blend
- Kale Chips (page 300) and almond milk
- Chia Pudding (page 300)
- 1–1½ ounces turkey or bison jerky
- ½–1 cup low-fat plain Greek yogurt with ½ cup fruit, ½ tablespoon chia seeds, 1 tablespoon oat bran, ½ ounce unsalted nuts
- Fruit smoothie (8 ounces soy milk, ½ cup fruit, 1–2 teaspoons chia seeds or flaxseeds, 1 tablespoon oat bran)
- Small apple or banana with 1 tablespoon peanut butter
- 2 tablespoons nuts (peanuts, almonds, pistachios, cashews, pecans, walnuts)
- 3 dried plums
- Lärabar
- Deviled Eggs (page 299)
- Toasted pita with Tzatziki Sauce (page 301)
- 1 cup edamame with olive oil and salt
- Herbal tea with 1 ounce dark chocolate (unless chocolate is a False Fix for you!)

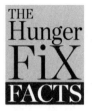

Chew on Chickpeas

Serotonin is essential for healthy functioning of the PFC, and low levels lead to worse mood, poorer social functioning, and depression and may even predispose you to physical problems like heart disease. Tryptophan, the "turkey" amino acid, is sometimes touted as a way to raise your serotonin. But many tryptophan foods also contain other amino acids in higher numbers, and the amino acids all compete for access into your brain. Tryptophan gets outnumbered and left behind.

One notable exception: the humble chickpea. Widely available cultivated versions of chickpeas have much more tryptophan than wild varieties. (Our ancestors probably noticed certain varieties made them feel good and bred them accordingly!) Sprinkle chickpeas on salad, snack on hummus (see the recipe on page 302), or add them to soup. Or just eat them cold, for a satisfying snack. In addition to their tryptophan content, chickpeas offer a nice dose of soluble fiber (4 grams per cup) to keep your blood sugar levels steady, lower your cholesterol, and help fight belly fat!

- Fresh Melon Granita (page 301)
- Hummus (page 302) with vegetable crudités
- Berry Yogurt Ice Pops (page 302)
- Cottage cheese with fruit
- Hard-cooked egg
- Low-sodium V8 juice with 1½ ounces trail mix
- Warm applesauce with high-fiber cereal
- Blue cheese dressing with vegetable crudités
- 1 ounce low-fat cheese and 1 whole grain rice cake
- Smoked almonds and iced green tea

CHAPTER 9

The Hunger Fix Recipes

THE HUNGER FIX RECIPES TAKE THEIR LEAD FROM the same ethic that I learned in Berkeley 30 years ago— high-quality ingredients and fresh whole foods, prepared simply. These meals, created by the chefs and dietitians at SPE Certified (the organization inspired by the Latin phrase Sanitas per Escam, or "Health through Food," which I introduced in Chapter 8), will be more delicious than any faux food False Fix you could ever encounter. Armed with all the new cooking skills you've learned in Chapter 8, these SPE Certified recipes should be a joy for you to create. Try to key in on the whole experience of cooking: selecting fresh ingredients at a farmers' market or local grocer, listening to music or drinking a glass of wine, dancing with your honey in the kitchen while the chicken bakes. As you get better at simple techniques, continue to challenge yourself. Make every part of cooking a sensual and dopamine-boosting experience, and you will fall in love with the whole process.

Remember: no fear. Nourish yourself and your family with the best foods on earth, a never-ending Healthy Fix. You can do this!

Smoothies

Smoothies are a quick and easy way to incorporate a balanced meal or snack into your day. The SPE nutritionists and I have created versatile recipes from a variety of milk and plant milks, fruits, fiber, and protein sources that can work for vegetarianism, lactose intolerance, and other dietary restrictions. Keep in mind that since you are training your palate to appreciate fewer sweet flavors, there is no added sugar in these smoothies. Also, if you have trouble finding a protein to add, you can omit it from the recipe, but be sure to have additional protein as part of the meal (around 20 grams of protein).

Milks

You can find many dairy and plant-based milks in the grocery store, including soy, almond, hemp, sunflower, and oat. Any unsweetened vanilla variety complements fruit smoothie flavors. Some plant and nut milks are shelf stable until opened and can be bought in bulk. We've listed milks and flavors that we feel work well; however, feel free to substitute other varieties that you may enjoy more. When shopping, look for unsweetened varieties with all natural ingredients.

Protein Sources

We incorporate several different protein sources to boost the total protein in the smoothie and make it an acceptable meal replacement. While we used tofu and nut butters as the plant-based protein sources in these recipes, you could also try powdered vegetable protein. We also use fat-free Greek yogurt and whey protein as animal-based protein boosters. In making the smoothies, you'll find that some work better with respect to flavor and texture. We put forth the combinations we found the best. For example, whey protein works well with cocoa powder. For the Tropical Smoothie, almost any combination works.

Fiber

To add fiber, we include the peels and skins of the fruits used in the smoothies whenever possible. You'll find that using the citrus peel simplifies preparation since you don't have to peel the fruit and it boosts the citrus flavor in the smoothie. We include ground flaxseed, chia seed, and nuts, which have the added benefit of healthy fats. Oat and wheat bran are also options; however, they do not contain as much fiber and healthy fats of some of the other choices.

Fruit

Fruit adds fiber and flavor to smoothies. Frozen fruit improves the texture and temperature and eliminates the need to add ice, which can water down the smoothie. (Just let the fruit sit for a few minutes to thaw, to spare your blender blade!) Fruits can be picked or bought in season and frozen so that in the winter you can have a smoothie of summer fruits. When bananas start to get soft, you can put them in the freezer to use anytime. If you can't freeze your own, there is a wide variety of frozen fruit available in the freezer sections of grocery stores.

Spirulina

Two of the smoothies include spirulina, a powdered algae that contains protein, B vitamins, beta-carotene, and iron. It also contains phenylalanine, a dopamine precursor. It's a powder that can be added to just about any smoothie if you are looking for the added nutrients. The flavor can be strong, so our recipes call for 1 teaspoon; however, you can add up to 1 tablespoon as you become more accustomed to the taste. You can find spirulina in health food stores.

The recipes below are for full meal portions and range from 350 to 450 calories. A half recipe can be made for a snack at 125 to 225 calories. To make the smoothies, ensure the fruit is frozen and combine all the ingredients in a blender and blend until smooth. Enjoy!

Strawberry Banana Smoothie

1 cup vanilla soy milk

$\frac{1}{2}$ medium banana

$\frac{3}{4}$ cup strawberries

1 tablespoon chia seeds

$\frac{1}{2}$ cup silken tofu

1 lemon wedge with skin

Makes 1$\frac{3}{4}$ cups

Per serving: 310 calories, 19 g protein, 33 g carbohydrate, 12 g total fat, 1 g saturated fat, 12 g fiber, 41 mg sodium

Berry Smoothie

1$\frac{1}{4}$ cups vanilla soy milk

$\frac{1}{4}$ cup blueberries

$\frac{1}{4}$ cup raspberries

$\frac{1}{4}$ cup blackberries

$\frac{1}{2}$ scoop (12 g) whey protein

1 tablespoon chia seeds

1 lemon wedge with skin

Makes 2 cups

Per serving: 293 calories, 23 g protein, 28 g carbohydrate, 10 g total fat, 1 g saturated fat, 13 g fiber, 60 mg sodium

Peanut Butter Banana Chocolate Smoothie

$\frac{3}{4}$ cup fat-free milk

1 medium banana

1 tablespoon peanut butter

1 tablespoon cocoa powder

1 tablespoon ground flaxseed

1 scoop (24 g) whey protein powder

Makes 1$\frac{3}{4}$ cups

Per serving: 423 calories, 33 g protein, 46 g carbohydrate, 13 g total fat, 3 g saturated fat, 7 g fiber, 123 mg sodium

Chocolate Cherry Almond Smoothie

$\frac{1}{2}$ cup almond milk

1 cup chopped cherries, pitted

1 tablespoon cocoa powder

$\frac{1}{2}$ ounce almonds, whole

1 scoop (24 g) whey protein powder

1 tablespoon ground flaxseed

Makes 1 serving (about 1$\frac{1}{4}$ cups)

Per serving: 348 calories, 25 g protein, 33 g carbohydrate, 13 g total fat, 2 g saturated fat, 8 g fiber, 130 mg sodium

Tropical Smoothie

$^3/_4$ cup vanilla soy milk

$^1/_2$ cup pineapple chunks

$^1/_2$ small orange with skin

$^1/_2$ medium banana

1 tablespoon unsweetened shredded coconut

1 scoop (24 g) whey protein powder

Makes 1 serving (about 2$^1/_4$ cups)

Per serving: 362 calories, 28 g protein, 44 g carbohydrate, 10 g total fat, 5 g saturated fat, 10 g fiber, 68 mg sodium

Variation: Use 1 cup fat-free Greek yogurt in place of whey protein.

Per serving: 386 calories, 29 g protein, 51 g carbohydrate, 8 g total fat, 5 g saturated fat, 10 g fiber, 93 mg sodium

Vegan Variation: To make this vegan, use $^1/_2$ cup silken tofu in place of whey protein powder.

Per serving: 359 calories, 18 g protein, 47 g carbohydrate, 13 g total fat, 5 g saturated fat, 11 g fiber, 37 mg sodium

Green Granny

1 cup vanilla soy milk

1 cup fat-free Greek yogurt

$^1/_2$ cup Granny Smith apple

12 green grapes

1–2 wedges of lime

1 teaspoon chia seeds

1–2 teaspoons spirulina

Makes 2$^1/_2$ cups

Per serving: 311 calories, 30 g protein, 34 g carbohydrate, 6 g total fat, 1 g saturated fat, 9 g fiber, 140 mg sodium

Green Monster

1 cup vanilla soy milk

1 cup fat-free Greek yogurt

1 medium kiwifruit

$\frac{1}{2}$ cup chopped honeydew melon

12 green grapes

1–2 wedges of lime

1 teaspoon chia seeds

1–2 teaspoons spirulina

$\frac{1}{2}$ teaspoon minced fresh ginger (optional)

4 mint leaves (optional)

Makes 2½ cups

Per serving: 347 calories, 30 g protein, 43 g carbohydrate, 7 g total fat, 1 g saturated fat, 10 g fiber, 140 mg sodium

Pomegranate Raspberry Banana Smoothie

$\frac{3}{4}$ cup vanilla soy milk

1 cup fat-free Greek yogurt

$\frac{1}{2}$ medium banana

$\frac{1}{4}$ cup pomegranate seeds

$\frac{1}{4}$ cup raspberries

1 teaspoon chia seeds

Makes about 2 cups

Per serving: 309 calories, 27 g protein, 39 g carbohydrate, 6 g total fat, 1 g saturated fat, 10 g fiber, 82 mg sodium

Variation: To make the smoothie vegetarian, use 1 cup silken tofu in place of Greek yogurt.

Per serving: 329 calories, 20 g protein, 38 g carbohydrate, 12 g total fat, 1 g saturated fat, 10 g fiber, 37 mg sodium

Variation: Use 1 scoop (24 g) of whey protein in place of the Greek yogurt.

Per serving: 300 calories, 28 g protein, 33 g carbohydrate, 7 g total fat, 1 g saturated fat, 10 g fiber, 66 mg sodium

Peach Mango Smoothie

1 cup vanilla soy milk

$\frac{1}{3}$ cup sliced peaches

$\frac{1}{3}$ cup chopped mango

$\frac{1}{4}$ small orange with skin

1 scoop (24 g) whey protein

1 tablespoon ground flaxseed

Makes 2½ cups

Per serving: 314 calories, 30 g protein, 28 g carbohydrate, 9 g total fat, 2 g saturated fat, 9 g fiber, 71 mg sodium

Apple Cinnamon Yogurt Smoothie

1 cup vanilla soy milk

1 apple (cooked and mashed, with skins, cooled)

1 tablespoon raisins, plumped in warm water

1 cup fat-free Greek yogurt

$\frac{1}{2}$ ounce almonds

1 tablespoon ground flaxseed

$\frac{1}{4}$ teaspoon cinnamon

Makes 2½ cups

Per serving: 452 calories, 32 g protein, 52 g carbohydrate, 14 g total fat, 1 g saturated fat, 12 g fiber, 90 mg sodium

Variation: To make this smoothie vegetarian, you can replace the Greek yogurt with ½ cup silken tofu.

Per serving: 441 calories, 22 g protein, 49 g carbohydrate, 19 g total fat, 2 g saturated fat, 13 g fiber, 42 mg sodium

Vinaigrettes and Marinades

If you get these basics down, you'll never want for a proper Hunger Fix dinner—you'll be able to whip up a savory lean protein and a refreshing salad in no time.

Balsamic Vinaigrette

$^2/_3$ cup balsamic vinegar

1 tablespoon Dijon mustard

1 teaspoon brown sugar

1 teaspoon salt

$^1/_2$ teaspoon ground black pepper

$^1/_3$ cup extra-virgin olive oil

In a large bowl, combine the vinegar, mustard, brown sugar, salt, and pepper. Whisk together until well incorporated. Stream in the oil, continually whisking. This vinaigrette can be refrigerated for up to a week. Whisk it again each time prior to using.

Makes 18 servings (18 tablespoons)

Per serving: 46 calories, 0 g protein, 2 g carbohydrate, 4 g total fat, 1 g saturated fat, 0 g fiber, 153 mg sodium

Variation: Roasted Garlic Vinaigrette: Mince 2 cloves roasted garlic and add to the vinaigrette. To roast garlic, preheat the oven to 350°F. Wrap peeled garlic cloves with a small sheet of foil. Roast for 20 to 25 minutes. The garlic should be soft and fragrant, but not burnt.

Per serving: 46 calories, 0 g protein, 2 g carbohydrate, 4 g total fat, 1 g saturated fat, 0 g fiber, 153 mg sodium

Asian Vinaigrette

- $1/3$ cup unseasoned rice wine vinegar
- 2 tablespoons lemon juice or lime juice
- 2 teaspoons sesame oil
- 1 teaspoon brown sugar
- $1/2$ teaspoon minced fresh ginger
- $1/4$ teaspoon salt
- $1/4$ teaspoon minced garlic
- $1/8$ teaspoon red pepper flakes

In a small bowl, whisk together the rice wine vinegar, lemon or lime juice, oil, brown sugar, ginger, salt, garlic, and red pepper flakes. Pour the mixture over the salad and mix until combined.

Makes 6 servings

Per serving: 20 calories, 0 g protein, 1 g carbohydrate, 2 g total fat, 0 g saturated fat, 0 g fiber, 99 mg sodium

Champagne Vinaigrette

- $2/3$ cup champagne vinegar
- 2 tablespoons lemon juice
- 1 teaspoon agave syrup
- $1/2$ teaspoon salt
- $1/2$ teaspoon ground white pepper
- $1/3$ cup extra-virgin olive oil (see note)

In a medium bowl, combine the vinegar, lemon juice, agave, salt, and pepper. Whisk together until well incorporated. Stream in the oil, continually whisking. This vinaigrette can be refrigerated for up to a week. Whisk it prior to using.

Makes 18 servings (18 tablespoons)

Per serving: 39 calories, 0 g protein, 0 g carbohydrate, 4 g total fat, 1 g saturated fat, 0 g fiber, 66 mg sodium

Note: Hazelnut or walnut oil can be substituted for a unique flavor.

Red Wine Vinaigrette

$^2/_3$ cup red wine vinegar

2 tablespoons lemon juice

1 tablespoon Dijon mustard

1 teaspoon agave syrup

$^1/_2$ teaspoon salt

$^1/_2$ teaspoon ground black pepper

$^1/_3$ cup extra-virgin olive oil

In a medium bowl, combine the vinegar, lemon juice, mustard, agave, salt, and pepper. Whisk together until well incorporated. Stream in the oil, continually whisking. This vinaigrette can be refrigerated for up to a week. Whisk it prior to using.

Makes 18 servings (18 tablespoons)

Per serving: 40 calories, 0 g protein, 1 g carbohydrate, 4 g total fat, 1 g saturated fat, 0 g fiber, 86 mg sodium

Smoky Cumin Lime Vinaigrette

$^1/_2$ cup red wine vinegar

$^1/_4$ cup olive oil

$^1/_4$ cup lime juice

$1^1/_2$ tablespoons toasted cumin seeds (see note)

1 teaspoon sugar

1 teaspoon salt

$^1/_2$ teaspoon red pepper flakes

In a small bowl, whisk together the vinegar, oil, lime juice, cumin, sugar, salt, and red pepper flakes. Pour over the salad and toss well.

Makes 16–18 servings (16–18 tablespoons)

Per serving: 73 calories, 0 g protein, 3 g carbohydrates, 7 g total fat, 1 g saturated fat, 0 g fiber, 299 mg sodium

Note: Toast the cumin in a small skillet over medium-high heat.

Seafood Marinades

Use with salmon, sole, cod, tilapia, shrimp, trout, tuna, or swordfish.

Lemon Caper Marinade

2 tablespoons olive oil

2 cloves garlic, minced

Juice and grated peel of 1 lemon

2 tablespoons capers

¼ teaspoon ground black pepper

Pinch of salt

Pinch of sugar

1 tablespoon chopped fresh parsley (optional)

In a small bowl, combine all of the ingredients and parsley (if using). Pour over the item being marinated. Let marinate for at least 15 minutes.

Makes enough for 1 pound of shrimp or fish

Per serving: 7 calories, 0 g protein, 0 g carbohydrate, 1 g total fat, 0 g saturated fat, 0 g fiber, 16 mg sodium

Lemon Pepper Marinade

2 tablespoons olive oil

2 cloves garlic, minced

Juice and grated peel of 1 lemon

½ teaspoon sea salt

½ teaspoon ground black pepper

Pinch of sugar

1 tablespoon chopped fresh parsley (optional)

In a small bowl, combine all of the ingredients and parsley (if using). Pour over the item being marinated. Let marinate for at least 15 minutes.

Makes enough for 1 pound of shrimp or fish

Per serving: 7 calories, 0 g protein, 0 g carbohydrate, 1 g total fat, 0 g saturated fat, 0 g fiber, 30 mg sodium

Hot and Spicy Marinade

2 tablespoons olive oil

2 tablespoons Tabasco sauce

2 tablespoons red wine vinegar

1 teaspoon red pepper flakes

2 cloves garlic, minced

1 teaspoon Dijon mustard

$\frac{1}{2}$ teaspoon sugar

$\frac{1}{2}$ teaspoon salt

$\frac{1}{4}$ teaspoon ground black pepper

In a small bowl, combine the oil, Tabasco sauce, vinegar, red pepper flakes, garlic, mustard, sugar, salt, and black pepper. Pour over the item being marinated. Let marinate for at least 15 minutes.

Makes enough for 1 pound of shrimp or fish

Per serving: 7 calories, 0 g protein, 0 g carbohydrate, 1 g total fat, 0 g saturated fat, 0 g fiber, 31 mg sodium

Miso Citrus Marinade

6 tablespoons orange juice (about 1 orange)

2 tablespoons lemon juice (about $\frac{1}{2}$ lemon)

1 tablespoon lime juice (about $\frac{1}{2}$ lime)

$\frac{1}{4}$ cup miso paste

$\frac{1}{4}$ cup reduced-sodium soy sauce

3 tablespoons rice wine vinegar

2 tablespoons packed brown sugar

$\frac{1}{2}$ tablespoon sesame oil

$\frac{1}{2}$ cup chopped scallions

$\frac{1}{2}$ cup chopped cilantro

2 tablespoons minced fresh ginger

2 cloves minced garlic

Pinch of salt

Pinch of ground black pepper

(continued)

In a large bowl, combine the juices, miso paste, soy sauce, vinegar, sugar, and oil. Mix the marinade until the sugar is dissolved and the miso paste is well incorporated. Mix in the scallions, cilantro, ginger, garlic, salt, and pepper to the marinade. Pour over the item being marinated. Let marinate for at least 15 minutes.

Makes enough for 2 pounds of shrimp or fish

Per serving: 9 calories, 0 g protein, 1 g carbohydrate, 1 g total fat, 0 g saturated fat, 0 g fiber, 97 mg sodium

Meat Marinades

These marinades are ideal for pork and other red meats.

Red Wine Marinade

 $\frac{1}{4}$ cup red wine

3 cloves garlic, minced

2 tablespoons chopped fresh rosemary (see note)

1 tablespoon chopped fresh thyme (see note)

2 teaspoons olive oil

 $\frac{1}{2}$ teaspoon salt

 $\frac{1}{2}$ teaspoon ground black pepper

In a small bowl, combine the red wine, garlic, rosemary, thyme, oil, salt, and pepper. Pour over the item being marinated. Let marinate for at least 15 minutes.

Makes enough for 1 pound of meat

Per serving: 4 calories, 0 g protein, 0 g carbohydrate, 0 g total fat, 0 g saturated fat, 0 g fiber, 30 mg sodium

Note: If using dried herbs, use half the amount of fresh herbs.

Steak Marinade

¼ cup red wine

2 cloves garlic, sliced

2 tablespoons chopped fresh ginger

2 tablespoons Worcestershire sauce

2 tablespoons reduced-sodium soy sauce

2 teaspoons brown sugar

½ teaspoon salt

In a bowl, combine the red wine, garlic, ginger, Worcestershire sauce, soy sauce, brown sugar, and salt. Pour over the steaks being marinated. Let marinate for at least 15 minutes.

Makes enough for 2 steaks

Per serving: 7 calories, 0 g protein, 1 g carbohydrate, 0 g total fat, 0 g saturated fat, 0 g fiber, 129 mg sodium

Teriyaki Marinade

½ cup reduced-sodium soy sauce

¼ cup pineapple juice (see note)

4 cloves garlic, minced

4 tablespoons minced fresh ginger

2 tablespoons miso paste (optional)

1 tablespoon brown sugar

1 teaspoon sesame oil

¼ teaspoon red pepper flakes

In a small bowl, combine the soy sauce, pineapple juice, garlic, ginger, miso paste (if using), brown sugar, sesame oil, and red pepper flakes. Pour over the item being marinated. Let marinate for at least 15 minutes.

Makes enough for 1 pound of meat

Per serving: 6 calories, 0 g protein, 1 g carbohydrate, 0 g total fat, 0 g saturated fat, 0 g fiber, 106 mg sodium

Note: If marinating chicken, replace the pineapple juice with ¼ cup orange juice.

Lunches

I know that most of you don't have the luxury of cooking at home for lunch, so we've created many recipes you can prepare in advance and take with you. Feel free to substitute these in for a light dinner, if desired.

Stage 1 Lunches

You'll find many soups in Stage 1. Soup is a food addict's best friend—hard to eat too much, very filling, and full of amazing nutrition. Soup can be heated up incredibly quickly to help you "eat around" a craving.

Chicken Salad with Greek Yogurt

$\frac{1}{4}$ cup fat-free Greek yogurt

2 tablespoons chopped celery

1 tablespoon parsley

1 tablespoon chopped fresh chives

1 teaspoon mayonnaise

$\frac{1}{2}$ teaspoon Dijon mustard

Pinch of salt

Pinch of ground black pepper

$1\frac{1}{2}$ cups cooked chicken

In a mixing bowl, combine the yogurt, celery, parsley, chives, mayonnaise, mustard, salt, and pepper. Add in the cooked chicken. Mix well.

Makes 2 servings

Per serving: 207 calories, 35 g protein, 2 g carbohydrates, 6 g total fat, 1g saturated fat, 0 g fiber, 268 mg sodium

Variations: Tuna Salad with Greek Yogurt: Substitute two 5-ounce cans of tuna packed in water for the chicken. **Egg Salad with Greek Yogurt:** Substitute 4 hard-cooked eggs for the chicken. Works best when the eggs are still warm.

Three Bean Salad

2 cups steamed wax beans or 1 can (15 ounces) wax beans,
   low sodium

2 cups steamed green beans or 1 can (15 ounces) green beans,
   low sodium

2 cups cooked kidney beans or 1 can (15 ounces) kidney beans,
   low sodium

2 cups cooked chickpeas or 1 can (15 ounces) chickpeas,
   low sodium

2 tablespoons olive oil

½ cup chopped onion (1 small onion)

1 clove garlic, minced

1 cup white vinegar

1 teaspoon sugar

1 teaspoon salt

½ teaspoon ground black pepper

In a large bowl, combine the wax beans, green beans, kidney beans,
and chickpeas. Heat the oil in a small skillet over medium-high heat.
Add the onion and garlic. Cook, stirring frequently, for 1 to 2 minutes.
Add the vinegar, sugar, salt, and pepper. Whisk together for 1 minute. Pour over the beans. Toss well.

Makes 6–8 servings (9 cups)

Per serving: 180 calories, 10 g protein, 32 g carbohydrate, 2 g total fat,
0 g saturated fat, 9 g fiber, 343 mg sodium

Crispy Tofu

1 package (10 ounces) extrafirm tofu, drained and sliced into
   2″ x 1″ pieces

3 cloves garlic, chopped

2 tablespoons lemon juice

2 tablespoons canola oil

½ teaspoon salt

½ teaspoon ground black pepper

(continued)

Preheat the oven to 400°F. Wrap the tofu in paper towels and set aside for 10 minutes. Line a baking dish with foil. In a small bowl, combine the garlic, lemon juice, canola oil, salt, and pepper. Place the tofu into the baking dish and coat on all sides with the mixture. Bake the tofu in the oven for 45 to 60 minutes, or until golden brown and crispy.

Makes 2 servings

Per serving: 211 calories, 15 g protein, 7 g carbohydrates, 14 g total fat, 2 g saturated fat, 2 g fiber, 596 mg sodium

Vegetable Soup

   2 teaspoons olive oil

   3 cloves garlic, minced

   1 medium onion, chopped

   1 cup chopped celery

   1 cup chopped carrots

   1 sprig fresh thyme or $\frac{1}{2}$ teaspoon dried thyme

   1 teaspoon paprika

   $1\frac{1}{2}$–2 quarts chicken or vegetable stock (see page 240)

   1 can (14 ounces) diced tomatoes (low or no sodium)

   1 cup chopped green beans

   1 can (7 ounces) corn or 1 cup fresh or frozen corn

   2 cups chopped spinach

   $\frac{1}{4}$ cup chopped parsley

   1 teaspoon salt

   $\frac{1}{2}$ teaspoon ground black pepper

Heat the oil in a large pot over medium-high heat. Add the garlic and onion. Cook, stirring frequently, for 1 to 2 minutes, or until softened. Add the celery, carrots, thyme, and paprika. Continue cooking for 5 to 10 minutes. Add $1\frac{1}{2}$ quarts of the stock and the tomatoes. Simmer for 10 minutes, or until the vegetables are softened. Add the green beans, corn, spinach, parsley. Add more stock if needed. Season the soup with the salt and pepper.

Makes 6 servings

Per serving: 98 calories, 6 g protein, 16 g carbohydrate, 2 g total fat, 0 g saturated fat, 4 g fiber, 687 mg sodium

Minestrone Soup

2 teaspoons olive oil

4 cloves garlic, minced

1 medium onion, chopped

4 medium carrots, chopped

4 ribs celery, chopped

2 medium tomatoes, chopped, or 1 can (14 ounces) diced
   tomatoes, no or low sodium

1 sprig fresh thyme or 1 teaspoon dried thyme

1 teaspoon salt

1½–2 quarts chicken or vegetable stock (see page 240)

1 cup soaked kidney beans or 1 can (15 ounces) kidney beans

1 small zucchini, chopped

1 small yellow squash, chopped

1 cup chopped parsley

2 tablespoons pesto (optional)

½ teaspoon red pepper flakes

¼ teaspoon ground black pepper

Heat the oil in a large pot over medium-high heat. Add the garlic and onion. Cook, stirring frequently, for 1 to 2 minutes, or until softened. Add the carrots and celery. Continue cooking for 5 minutes. Next, add the tomatoes, thyme, and salt. After a few minutes, add 1 quart of the stock and the kidney beans (if using canned kidney beans, add at the end of the recipe). Simmer for 20 minutes, or until the beans and vegetables are tender. Add more stock if needed. Add the zucchini, yellow squash, parsley, and pesto (if using). Season the minestrone with the red pepper flakes and black pepper.

Makes 8 servings

Per serving: 93 calories, 6 g protein, 15 g carbohydrate, 2 g total fat,
0 g saturated fat, 4 g fiber, 481 mg sodium

Chicken Vegetable Soup

2 teaspoons olive oil

4 cloves garlic, minced

1 medium onion, chopped

4 large carrots chopped

4 ribs celery, chopped

1 large parsnip, chopped

1 package (10 ounces) white button mushrooms, sliced

1½–2 quarts chicken or vegetable stock (see page 240)

4 cups diced cooked chicken

½ cup sliced scallions

¼ cup chopped parsley

2 teaspoons salt

¼ teaspoon ground black pepper

Heat the oil in a large pot over medium-high heat. Add the garlic and onion. Cook, stirring frequently, for 1 to 2 minutes, or until softened. Add the carrots, celery, parsnip, and mushrooms. Continue cooking for 5 to 10 minutes. Add the stock and bring to a boil. Reduce the heat to low and simmer for 10 minutes, or until the vegetables are softened. Add the chicken, scallions, parsley, salt, and pepper. Continue to cook until the chicken is heated through.

Makes 8 servings

Per serving: 193 calories, 27 g protein, 13 g carbohydrate, 4 g total fat, 1 g saturated fat, 3 g fiber, 517 mg sodium

Note: This soup can be made vegetarian by using vegetable stock and adding 14 ounces chopped, extrafirm tofu with the scallions and parsley.

Stage 2 Lunches

I strived to keep Stage 2 lunches simple yet flavored with a bit more variety and intrigue. Again, soups are a huge benefit to quelling any False Fix urges—they fill you up quickly and are very hard to overeat to an unhealthful degree. Your PFC is starting to become addicted to those Healthy Fixes. Keep practicing!

Smoky Tomato Bean Soup

  2 teaspoons olive oil

  1 medium onion, chopped

  4 cloves garlic, roasted (see note)

  1 can (28 ounces) low or no-sodium whole tomatoes or $1\frac{1}{2}$ pounds
     chopped fresh tomatoes

  1 teaspoon smoked paprika

  1 teaspoon salt

  Pinch of sugar

  $1-1\frac{1}{2}$ quarts chicken or vegetable stock (see page 240)

  $1\frac{1}{2}$ cups cooked white beans or 1 can (14 ounces) low- or
     no-sodium white beans, drained and rinsed

  $\frac{1}{4}$ cup chopped cilantro

  $\frac{1}{2}-1$ teaspoon Tabasco chipotle pepper sauce

Heat the oil in a large pot over medium-high heat. Cook the onion, stirring frequently, for 1 to 2 minutes, or until softened. Add the roasted garlic, tomatoes, smoked paprika, salt, and sugar. After 5 to 7 minutes, add 1 quart of the stock and the beans to the pot. Bring to a simmer and cook for 20 minutes. Remove the pot from the heat and puree using a stick blender, adding more stock if necessary to blend. Season the soup with the cilantro and chipotle sauce.

Makes 6 servings

Per serving: 123 calories, 8 g protein, 20 g carbohydrate, 2 g total fat, 0 g saturated fat, 5 g fiber, 537 mg sodium

Note: Preheat the oven to 350°F. Wrap peeled garlic cloves with a small sheet of foil. Roast for 20 to 25 minutes. The garlic should be soft and fragrant, but not burnt.

Turkey Chili

2 teaspoons olive oil

4 cloves garlic, minced

1 medium onion, chopped

1 pound ground turkey (see note)

2 teaspoons ground cumin

2 teaspoons ground cinnamon

$\frac{1}{4}$–1 teaspoon ground red pepper

$\frac{1}{4}$–1 teaspoon chili powder

1 large can (28 ounces) crushed tomatoes

$1\frac{1}{2}$ cups corn or 1 can (12 ounces) corn

$1\frac{1}{2}$ cups cooked black beans or 1 can (14 ounces) black beans, rinsed and drained

$1\frac{1}{2}$ cups cooked red kidney beans or 1 can (14 ounces) red kidney beans, rinsed and drained

1 medium red bell pepper, chopped

1 jalapeño pepper, chopped (optional)

1 teaspoon salt

$\frac{1}{2}$ teaspoon ground black pepper

$\frac{1}{4}$ cup chopped cilantro

Heat the oil in a large pot over medium-high heat. Add the garlic and onion. Cook, stirring frequently, for 1 to 2 minutes, or until softened. Add the ground turkey. Brown the turkey in the pot, being careful not to separate the turkey into small bits. Add the cumin, cinnamon, red pepper, and chili powder (see note). Add the tomatoes and bring the chili to a simmer. Add the corn, beans, bell pepper, and jalapeño pepper, if desired. Season with salt and black pepper. Return the chili to a simmer. Remove from the heat. Garnish with the cilantro.

Makes 6 servings

Per serving: 360 calories, 27 g protein, 43 g carbohydrate, 9 g total fat, 2 g saturated fat, 12 g fiber, 478 mg sodium

Note: You can use textured vegetable protein (TVP) in place of turkey to make this a vegetarian chili. For those who want a spicier chili, add more red pepper and chili powder a little at a time, tasting to avoid overly spicing the dish.

Crispy Tofu Carrot Salad

$\frac{1}{2}$ teaspoon salt, divided

6 large carrots, sliced on the bias into 2" x 1" pieces

20 ounces Crispy Tofu (page 259)

2 avocados, sliced

$\frac{1}{2}$ cup chopped cilantro

$\frac{1}{4}$ cup chopped scallions

2 teaspoons olive oil

1–2 tablespoons lime juice

Pinch of ground black pepper

In a large pot, bring water to a boil and add $\frac{1}{4}$ teaspoon of the salt. Submerge the carrots into the boiling water for 3 minutes. Strain the pot and run the carrots under cool water. While the Crispy Tofu and carrots are still warm, combine in a large bowl the tofu, carrots, avocados, cilantro, scallions, olive oil, lime juice, remaining $\frac{1}{4}$ teaspoon salt, and pepper.

Makes 4 servings

Per serving: 392 calories, 17 g protein, 24 g carbohydrates, 27 g total fat, 3 g saturated fat, 10 g fiber, 973 mg sodium

Roasted Turkey Breast

1 turkey breast, 2–3 pounds

1 teaspoon salt

1 teaspoon ground black pepper

Preheat the oven to 325°F. Place the turkey breast, skin side up, in a large roasting pan with sides. Season the turkey skin with salt and pepper. Roast for 1$\frac{1}{2}$ to 2 hours (longer for a larger breast), or until a thermometer inserted in the thickest portion registers 170°F and the juices run clear. Let the turkey sit for 10 minutes prior to carving. Save the bones for poultry stock (see page 240).

Makes 8–10 servings

Per serving: 363 calories, 55 g protein, 0 g carbohydrate, 14 g total fat, 4 g saturated fat, 0 g fiber, 383 mg sodium

Rhode Island Chowder

2 teaspoons olive oil

4 cloves garlic, minced

1 medium onion, chopped

4 ribs celery, chopped

4 large carrots, chopped

1 small fennel bulb, chopped (optional)

½ pound Red Bliss potatoes (4 small), washed and chopped

1 quart water or shrimp stock (see page 240)

1 cup clam juice

3 pounds clams, washed and steamed and removed from shells,
    or 3 cans (6.5 ounces each) clams

½ cup chopped parsley

¼ cup chopped fresh chives

1 tablespoon lemon juice

1 teaspoon smoked paprika

½ teaspoon ground black pepper

Heat the oil in a large pot over medium-high heat. Add the garlic and onion. Cook, stirring frequently, for 1 to 2 minutes, or until softened. Add the celery, carrots, and fennel (if using). Lower to medium heat and cook for 5 to 10 minutes. Add the potatoes, water or stock, and clam juice. Bring to a boil. Reduce the heat to a simmer and cook for 20 minutes, or until the vegetables are tender. Add the clams, parsley, chives, lemon juice, paprika, and pepper. Remove from the heat after 1 minute.

Makes 6 servings

Per serving: 163 calories, 14 g protein, 20 g carbohydrate, 3 g total fat, 0 g saturated fat, 4 g fiber, 792 mg sodium

Lentil Soup

1 cup dried lentils

2 teaspoons olive oil

2 cloves garlic, minced

1 medium onion, chopped

2 large carrots, chopped

2 ribs celery, chopped

2 cups cooked, cubed ham

1 cup chopped tomatoes or 1 can (14 ounces) low-sodium,
   diced tomatoes

1 bay leaf

$\frac{1}{2}$ teaspoon fresh thyme

$\frac{1}{4}$ teaspoon fresh rosemary

$1\frac{1}{2}$–2 quarts no-sodium chicken or vegetable stock (see page 240)

$\frac{1}{2}$ teaspoon ground black pepper

Pinch of salt

$\frac{1}{4}$ cup chopped parsley

In a pot, rinse and soak the lentils for at least 2 hours in cold,
unsalted water. Rinse, strain, and set aside. Heat the oil in a large pot
over medium-high heat. Add the garlic and onion. Cook, stirring frequently, for 1 to 2 minutes, or until translucent. Add the carrots and
celery. Continue to cook for 5 to 10 minutes, or until softened. Add
the ham, tomatoes, bay leaf, thyme, and rosemary. Add $1\frac{1}{2}$ quarts of
the stock. Simmer on low heat for 20 to 30 minutes, or until the lentils are al dente (see note). Add more stock if necessary. Season the
soup with the pepper and salt. Garnish with the parsley.

Makes 8 servings

Per serving: 249 calories, 21 g protein, 22 g carbohydrate, 9 g total fat,
3 g saturated fat, 9 g fiber, 845 mg sodium

Note: The lentils will continue to absorb water, so it is better to undercook them.

Roasted Beets

1 pound fresh, small beets (6 small beets)

$\frac{1}{3}$ cup kosher salt (see note)

1 teaspoon olive oil

$\frac{1}{4}$ teaspoon salt

$\frac{1}{4}$ teaspoon ground black pepper

Preheat the oven to 400°F. Trim the greens from the beets and wash well (see note). Leave the skin on. Spread the kosher salt over the bottom of a 9" x 9" baking dish. Place a piece of foil in the baking dish over the kosher salt (see note). Add the beets to the baking dish and fold the foil over the beets. Roast the beets in the oven for 45 minutes. Larger beets will take more time to roast and baby beets will take less time. Beets should be tender when done.

Once the beets have cooled, remove the skin and quarter the beets. Heat the oil in a large skillet over medium-high heat. Add the beets. Cook, stirring frequently, to reheat the beets. Season with the salt and pepper. The beets are now ready to serve or can be saved for a salad.

Makes 4 servings

Per serving: 59 calories, 2 g protein, 11 g carbohydrates, 1 g total fat, 0 g saturated fat, 3 g fiber, 236 mg sodium

Note: Beet greens are very nutritious and should not be discarded. They can be washed and used in place of kale or Swiss chard. Having kosher salt on the bottom of the baking dish will prevent the beets from burning while roasting in the oven. Make sure the foil for the baking dish is large enough to be folded over and cover the beets.

Broccoli Cheddar Soup with Chicken

2 teaspoons olive oil

2 cloves garlic, minced

1 small onion, chopped

1½ quarts chicken stock (see page 240)

6 cups broccoli florets (2 bunches or 4 crowns)

½ cup reduced-fat, sharp Cheddar cheese

2 cups cooked chicken

¼ teaspoon salt

¼ teaspoon ground black pepper

Dash of ground nutmeg

Heat the oil in a large pot over medium-high heat. Add the garlic and onion. Cook, stirring frequently, for 4 to 5 minutes, or until soft. Add the chicken stock and bring to a boil. Add the broccoli and cover the pot. Reduce the heat to medium and simmer for 5 to 7 minutes. With a stick blender or a regular blender, puree the soup. Stir in the cheese. Add the chicken, salt, pepper, and nutmeg.

Makes 4 servings

Per serving: 245 calories, 33 g protein, 13 g carbohydrate, 8 g total fat, 2 g saturated fat, 4 g fiber, 542 mg sodium

Note: This soup can be frozen. This soup can be made vegetarian by replacing the chicken stock with vegetable stock (see page 240) and using tofu instead of chicken. Before pureeing soup, add 14 ounces (1 package) of silken tofu into the soup.

Chickpea Salad

1 can (14 ounces) chickpeas, rinsed and drained

2 cups chopped tomatoes

1½ cups chopped cucumber

2 tablespoons chopped red onion

½ teaspoon salt

½ teaspoon ground black pepper

Pinch of sugar

¼ cup red wine vinegar

2 tablespoons extra-virgin olive oil

¼ cup fresh, thinly sliced basil leaves

In a medium bowl, combine the chickpeas, tomatoes, cucumber, and red onion. Season the salad with the salt, pepper, and sugar. Pour the vinegar and oil over the salad. Toss well. Garnish with the basil.

Makes 6 servings (6 cups)

Per serving: 167 calories, 7 g protein, 22 g carbohydrate, 6 g total fat, 1 g saturated fat, 6 g fiber, 206 mg sodium

Hearty Southwestern Chicken Stew

1 tablespoon olive oil

2 large cloves garlic, minced

1 cup chopped celery

1 cup chopped carrot

$\frac{1}{2}$ cup chopped onion

2 quarts chicken stock (see page 240)

1 can (14 ounces) diced tomatoes

3 cups chopped cooked chicken

1 cup canned black beans, rinsed and drained

1 cup frozen or canned corn

$\frac{1}{2}$ cup chopped red bell pepper

$\frac{1}{2}$ cup sliced okra

$\frac{1}{2}$ cup fat-free Greek yogurt

2 tablespoons lemon juice

1–2 teaspoons chipotle-flavored hot sauce or 2 teaspoons
     smoked paprika

$\frac{1}{2}$ teaspoon ground black pepper

$\frac{1}{4}$ teaspoon salt

Heat the oil in a large pot over medium-high heat. Add the garlic,
celery, carrot, and onion. Cook, stirring frequently, for 5 to 7 minutes,
or until soft. Add the chicken stock and tomatoes (with juice). Bring
to a boil. Reduce the heat and simmer for 10 minutes. Add the
chicken, black beans, corn, bell pepper, and okra. Take 1 cup chicken
stock from the stew and pour into a small bowl. Slowly add the
reserved stock to the Greek yogurt, constantly stirring. This will
allow you to add the yogurt into the soup without lumps forming.
Once the stock and yogurt are fully combined, add the yogurt mixture back into the soup. Return to a simmer and add more stock if
necessary. Season the dish with lemon juice, hot sauce or paprika,
black pepper, and salt.

Makes 6 servings

Per serving: 256 calories, 32 g protein, 23 g carbohydrate, 5 g total fat,
1 g saturated fat, 6 g fiber, 594 mg sodium

Sweet and Spicy Slaw

4–5 cups thinly sliced green cabbage ($\frac{1}{2}$ head of cabbage)

1 cup chopped red bell pepper

1 cup chopped cucumber

1 cup grated carrot

1 cup chickpeas, drained

$\frac{1}{2}$ cup chopped pineapple

$\frac{1}{2}$ cup chopped mango

$\frac{1}{4}$ cup chopped cilantro

$\frac{1}{4}$ cup chopped scallions

$\frac{1}{4}$ cup chopped fresh mint

$\frac{1}{4}$ cup peanuts

6 tablespoons Smoky Cumin Lime Vinaigrette (page 253)

In a large mixing bowl, combine the cabbage, bell pepper, cucumber, carrot, chickpeas, pineapple, mango, cilantro, scallions, and mint. In a medium skillet over medium heat, roast the peanuts until golden and fragrant. Set aside. Whisk the vinaigrette and pour over the slaw. Mix well. Garnish with the roasted peanuts.

Makes 6 servings (8 cups)

Per serving: 204 calories, 5 g protein, 24 g carbohydrates, 11 g total fat, 1 g saturated fat, 5 g fiber, 444 mg sodium

Variation: For an Asian slaw, combine a shredded head of cabbage, 1 cup sliced scallions, and $\frac{1}{2}$ cup chopped fresh cilantro in a large bowl. Add 8 tablespoons of the Asian Vinaigrette (page 252), mix, and refrigerate for at least 15 minutes. Top with $\frac{1}{2}$ cup toasted sliced almonds and $\frac{1}{4}$ cup toasted sesame seeds.

Stage 3 Lunches

By this point, you are such a pro, you could probably write these recipes! Take a look to see how to expand your culinary skills even further. Use these recipes as a springboard for your own creations. As long as you strive to include a variety of vegetables and spices in your foods, your epigenetic changes continue to get stronger with every meal.

Gazpacho

$\frac{1}{2}$ piece stale bread

$\frac{1}{4}$ cup warm water

3 cloves garlic

$1\frac{1}{2}$ teaspoons salt

2 tablespoons cumin seeds

3 pound tomatoes, cored and chopped

2 tablespoons olive oil

1 teaspoon sugar

$\frac{1}{3}$ cup sherry vinegar (such as Pedro Ximénez)

$\frac{1}{4}$ teaspoon ground red pepper

$\frac{1}{4}$ cup red bell pepper, diced

$\frac{1}{4}$ cup yellow bell pepper, diced

$\frac{1}{2}$ cup cucumber, diced

$\frac{1}{2}$ avocado, sliced (optional)

Soak the bread in the warm water for 3 minutes. Smash the garlic cloves with a large knife. Mash the cloves together with the salt, using a fork or the side of the knife blade. Once the garlic starts breaking down, add the cumin seeds. Squeeze the water from the bread and add the bread to the garlic, then continue mashing until a paste forms. Process the tomatoes in a food processor in batches of three. After the tomatoes have been processed for a minute, add one-third of the garlic paste, olive oil, sugar, and vinegar. Process until smooth, then transfer to a large bowl. Do the same for the next

(continued)

two batches. Season with the ground red pepper. Chill the soup for at least 1 hour. Garnish with the chopped peppers, cucumber, and avocado (if desired) before serving.

Makes 8 servings (8 cups)

Per serving: 82 calories, 2 g protein, 10 g carbohydrate, 4 g total fat, 1 g saturated fat, 3 g fiber, 463 mg sodium

Waldorf Salad

¼ cup raisins

2 tablespoons fat-free Greek yogurt

2 teaspoons mayonnaise

1 tablespoon lemon juice

4 large ribs celery, chopped

2 medium apples (red delicious), chopped

¼ cup roasted walnuts, chopped

Into a small bowl, put the raisins and cover with hot (not boiling) water. Let the raisins stand for 5 minutes and then drain. The raisins should be nice and plump at this point. Set aside. In a small bowl, combine the yogurt, mayonnaise, and lemon juice. Mix well. In a medium bowl, combine the celery, apples, and raisins. Pour in the yogurt mixture. Toss well. Garnish with the walnuts.

Makes 2 servings

Per serving: 309 calories, 5 g protein, 46 g carbohydrate, 14 g total fat, 2 g saturated fat, 9 g fiber, 136 mg sodium

Mushroom Soup

1 tablespoon olive oil

2 shallots, chopped

2 cloves garlic, minced

1 small onion, chopped

32 ounces fresh mushrooms, chopped (see note)

2 cups chicken or vegetable stock (see page 240)

1 tablespoon balsamic vinegar

8 cups 1% milk, divided

$\frac{1}{2}$ cup unbleached or all-purpose flour

1 teaspoon salt

Pinch of ground black pepper

$\frac{1}{4}$ cup chopped parsley

$\frac{1}{4}$ cup chopped chives (optional)

Heat the oil in a large stockpot over medium heat. Add the shallots, garlic, and onion. Cook, stirring frequently, for 2 to 3 minutes. Then add the mushrooms and a pinch of salt. Cook for 5 to 10 minutes, or until most of the moisture has cooked off. Add the stock, vinegar, and 7 cups of the milk to the pot. Bring the soup to a simmer. In a small bowl, add the flour to the remaining cup of cold milk to make a slurry. Whisk until there are no more lumps. Add the slurry to the soup. Bring the soup to a simmer for 5 minutes, until it thickens, but do not allow the soup to boil. Season with the salt and pepper. Garnish with the parsley and chives (if using) before serving.

Makes 6 servings (12 cups)

Per serving: 252 calories, 17 g protein, 35 g carbohydrates, 6 g total fat, 2 g saturated fat, 2 g fiber, 596 mg sodium

Note: One or a combination of different mushroom varieties, such as crimini, shiitake, oyster, chanterelle, or porcini, can be used.

Swordfish Kebabs

2 tablespoons lemon juice

1 clove garlic, chopped

1 teaspoon olive oil

¼ teaspoon salt

¼ teaspoon pepper

1 pound swordfish or tuna, cut into 1" cubes

2 small yellow squash, chopped into 1" pieces

2 small zucchini, chopped into 1" pieces

10 ounces button mushrooms (1 package), stems trimmed

1 medium red onion, chopped into 1" pieces

Pinch of salt

Pinch of ground black pepper

2 tablespoons lemon juice

In a medium bowl, combine the lemon juice, garlic, olive oil, salt, and pepper. Add the swordfish and mix so that the fish is well coated in the marinade. Marinate for 15 minutes. If using wooden skewers, soak them in water for a few minutes. Once soaked, place the squash, zucchini, mushrooms, onion, and fish on skewers so that they are distributed evenly. Lightly spray the skewers with nonstick cooking spray. Grill on all sides until the vegetables are softened and the swordfish is cooked through. Season the kebabs with the salt, pepper, and fresh lemon juice before serving.

Makes 3–4 servings

Per serving: 255 calories, 30 g protein, 11 g carbohydrate, 11 g total fat, 2 g saturated fat, 3 g fiber, 370 mg sodium

Cucumber and Lentil Salad

Salad

1 cup uncooked brown rice or 2½ cups cooked brown rice

⅔ cup uncooked lentils or 2 cups cooked lentils

2 cups chopped seedless cucumber (about 2 medium)

1 cup grated carrot (about 2 medium)

2 tablespoons chopped fresh dill (optional)

2 tablespoons chopped fresh chives (optional)

Vinaigrette

½ cup rice wine vinegar

2 tablespoons olive oil

1 teaspoon salt

1 teaspoon sugar

½ teaspoon ground black pepper

To make the salad: If using dried rice and lentils, cook the rice and lentils according to the package instructions. (It is best to slightly undercook rice and lentils so that they better absorb the vinaigrette.) In a large bowl, combine the cooked rice and lentils with the cucumber, carrot, and herbs (if desired).

To make the vinaigrette: In a small bowl, whisk together the vinegar, oil, salt, sugar, and pepper. Pour over the salad and toss well.

Makes 6 servings (6 cups)

Per serving: 249 calories, 8 g protein, 40 g carbohydrates, 6 g total fat, 1 g saturated fat, 8 g fiber, 410 mg sodium

Chicken Escarole Soup

2 teaspoons olive oil

4 cloves garlic, minced

1 medium onion, chopped

2 large carrots, chopped

2 ribs celery, chopped

2 quarts chicken or vegetable stock (see page 240)

4 cups diced cooked chicken

4 packed cups washed and chopped escarole

1½ cups cooked cannellini beans or 1 can (14 ounces) cannellini
   beans

¼ cup chopped parsley

1 tablespoon lemon juice

2 teaspoons salt

¼ teaspoon ground black pepper

¼ teaspoon red pepper flakes

Heat the oil in a large pot over medium-high heat. Add the garlic and
onion. Cook, stirring frequently, for 1 to 2 minutes, or until softened.
Add the carrots and celery. Continue cooking for 5 to 10 minutes.
Add the stock and bring to a boil. Reduce the heat and simmer for
10 minutes, or until the vegetables are softened. Add the chicken,
escarole, beans, and parsley. Remove the soup from the heat to
avoid overcooking the escarole. Season the soup with the lemon
juice, salt, black pepper, and red pepper flakes.

Makes 8 servings (12 cups)

Per serving: 201 calories, 28 g protein, 12 g carbohydrate, 4 g total fat,
1 g saturated fat, 4 g fiber, 530 mg sodium

Note: This soup can be made vegetarian by using vegetable stock and adding 14 ounces chopped,
extrafirm tofu with the beans.

Italian Farro Salad

1 cup dry farro or 2½ cups cooked farro

¼ cup dry lentils or ¾ cup cooked lentils

1 teaspoon olive oil

1 clove garlic, minced

½ cup chopped zucchini

½ cup chopped yellow squash

Pinch of salt

½ cup quartered cherry or grape tomatoes

½ cup (2 ounces) fresh mozzarella cheese, sliced

¼ cup chopped olives

¼ cup thinly sliced fresh basil

2 tablespoons lemon juice

4 tablespoons Roasted Garlic Vinaigrette (page 251)

Cook the farro and lentils according to package directions. (Farro can be a bit underdone for this salad so it better absorbs the vinaigrette.) In a skillet, heat the oil over medium-high heat. Add the garlic, zucchini, yellow squash, and pinch of salt. Cook for 5 minutes. In a large bowl, combine the cooked vegetables with the farro, lentils, tomatoes, cheese, olives, basil, and lemon juice. Whisk the vinaigrette and pour over the salad. Toss well and serve.

Makes 4 servings (4 cups)

Per serving: 309 calories, 13 g protein, 43 g carbohydrates, 10 g total fat, 2 g saturated fat, 9 g fiber, 280 mg sodium

Miso Citrus Salmon

6 tablespoons orange juice (about 1 orange)

¼ cup miso paste

¼ cup reduced-sodium soy sauce

3 tablespoons rice wine vinegar

2 tablespoons lemon juice (about ½ lemon)

1 tablespoon lime juice (about ½ lime)

2 tablespoons brown sugar

½ tablespoon sesame oil

½ cup chopped scallions

½ cup chopped cilantro

2 tablespoons minced fresh ginger

2 cloves garlic, minced

Pinch of salt

Pinch of ground black pepper

2 pounds salmon fillet

Preheat the oven to 350°F. In a large bowl, combine the orange juice, miso paste, soy sauce, vinegar, lemon juice, lime juice, sugar, and oil. Mix the marinade until the sugar is dissolved and the miso paste is well incorporated. Mix the scallions, cilantro, ginger, garlic, salt, and pepper into the marinade. Pour the marinade into a baking dish. Place the salmon in the baking dish with the skin side up and let stand for 15 minutes. Then, turn the fish over so that the skin side is down. Bake the salmon 25 to 30 minutes, or until the flesh is opaque.

Makes 5 servings (This dish uses 2 pounds of salmon because it works well for leftovers)

Per serving: 266 calories, 36 g protein, 1 g carbohydrates, 12 g total fat, 2 g saturated fat, 0 g fiber, 177 mg sodium

Variation: Replace all but the salmon with the Lemon Caper, Lemon Pepper, or Hot and Spicy Marinades (pages 254–255). Substitute 1 pound of another white fish.

Beef Barley Soup

2 teaspoons olive oil

1 pound lean beef (sirloin or chuck), chopped into 1" pieces

4 cloves garlic, sliced

1 medium onion, chopped

1 package (10 ounces) mushrooms, quartered

½ cup dried barley

1½–2 quarts beef stock (see page 240) or low-sodium beef stock

4 ribs celery, chopped

4 large carrots, chopped

1 tablespoon Worcestershire sauce

1 tablespoon balsamic vinegar

2 cups fresh or frozen peas

½ cup chopped parsley

1 teaspoon salt

½ teaspoon ground black pepper

Heat the oil in a large pot over medium-high heat. Add the beef and sauté until browned. Add the garlic and onion. Cook until the onions have softened. Add the mushrooms. Cook, stirring frequently, for 5 minutes. Next, add the barley and 1½ quarts beef stock. Bring the soup to a boil and reduce the heat to low. Cover the pot and simmer for 20 to 25 minutes, or until the barley is mostly cooked (see note). Add the celery, carrots, Worcestershire sauce, and vinegar. Simmer for 15 minutes. Once the carrots and celery are tender, add the peas, parsley, and more beef stock if necessary. Season the soup with the salt and pepper.

Makes 6 servings (9 cups)

Per serving: 279 calories, 26 g protein, 31 g carbohydrate, 6 g total fat, 2 g saturated fat, 7 g fiber, 716 mg sodium

Note: The barley should double in size when cooked.

Asian Shrimp Noodle Salad

3 tablespoons low-sodium soy sauce

3 tablespoons rice wine vinegar

1 tablespoon chili paste

1 tablespoon natural peanut butter

1 teaspoon sesame oil

1 large clove garlic, chopped

2 teaspoon minced fresh ginger

$\frac{1}{4}$ teaspoon red pepper flakes

$\frac{1}{2}$ pound shrimp, peeled and deveined

1 cup sliced carrot

$\frac{1}{4}$ cup sliced shiitake mushrooms

1 cup sugar snap peas, trimmed

1 cup sliced red bell pepper

1 bundle soba noodles (about 3 ounces)

$\frac{1}{4}$ cup chopped cilantro

$\frac{1}{4}$ cup sliced scallion

$\frac{1}{4}$ cup roasted peanuts

4 cups thinly sliced Napa cabbage

Start a pot of water to boil for the soba noodles. In a small bowl, whisk together the soy sauce, vinegar, chili paste, and peanut butter and set aside for later. In a large skillet over medium-high heat, heat the sesame oil. Cook the garlic, ginger, and red pepper flakes for 1 to 2 minutes. Add the shrimp and cook a minute on each side. Remove the shrimp from the pan and set aside. Add the carrot and mushrooms to the skillet and cook for 3 minutes. Add the sugar snaps and bell pepper and cook another 2 to 3 minutes. Once the water is boiling, cook the soba noodles as directed and add them to the skillet. Add the chili paste mixture and shrimp and cook for 2 to 3 minutes, stirring frequently. Remove from the heat and add the cilantro, scallions, and peanuts. Serve over the cabbage.

Makes 2–3 servings

Per serving: 493 calories, 36 g protein, 59 g carbohydrate, 15 g total fat, 2 g saturated fat, 10 g fiber, 1260 mg sodium

Dinners

Once you get comfortable with Stage 1 Dinners as your default evening meal, you'll be prepared for any "dangerous" food situation—and you'll also be ready to spread your wings in Stages 2 and 3. And your taste buds will be thankful!

Stage 1 Dinners

Stage 1 dinners are very basic—a lean protein with a vegetable—for a reason. I want to get your brain to see this Healthy Fix as the template for a Hunger Fix meal. (No grains at night, if you can avoid them.)

Roasted Butternut Squash

1 small butternut squash (about 1 pound), peeled, seeded, and
    cubed into $\frac{1}{2}$" pieces
1 tablespoon olive oil
1 tablespoon minced fresh ginger
$\frac{1}{4}$ teaspoon ground cinnamon
$\frac{1}{4}$ teaspoon ground nutmeg
$\frac{1}{4}$ teaspoon salt

Preheat the oven to 400°F. In a baking dish or pan, add the squash, oil, ginger, cinnamon, nutmeg, and salt. Toss well. Roast for 20 minutes, or until the squash is tender.

Makes 6 servings

Per serving: 73 calories, 1 g protein, 11 g carbohydrate, 4 g total fat, 1 g saturated fat, 2 g fiber, 151 mg sodium

Greek Salad

1 medium red bell pepper, chopped into 1″ pieces

1 medium green bell pepper, chopped into 1″ pieces

1 cup chopped tomatoes

1 cup chopped cucumber

½ cup chopped red onion

½ cup pitted kalamata olives

¼ cup chopped parsley

2 tablespoons Red Wine Vinaigrette (page 253)

¼ cup crumbled feta cheese

In a large bowl, combine the bell peppers, tomatoes, cucumber, red onion, olives, and parsley. Whisk or shake the vinaigrette well and drizzle over the salad. Toss well. Garnish with the feta cheese just before serving.

Makes 2 servings

Per serving: 207 calories, 6 g protein, 18 g carbohydrate, 13 g total fat, 4 g saturated fat, 5 g fiber, 521 mg sodium

Wilted Swiss Chard

1 bunch Swiss chard (12–16 ounces)

2 teaspoons olive oil

1 clove garlic, sliced

2 tablespoons rice wine vinegar

¼ teaspoon salt

¼ teaspoon ground black pepper

Wash the chard well and trim the fibrous ends. Heat the olive oil in a large skillet over medium-high heat and cook the garlic for 1 to 2 minutes. Add the chard and vinegar to the skillet. The chard will start wilting quickly. As soon as the chard is almost all wilted, remove it from the heat and season it with the salt and pepper.

Makes 3 servings

Per serving: 55 calories, 2 g protein, 6 g carbohydrate, 3 g total fat, 0 g saturated fat, 2 g fiber, 331 mg sodium

Stage 2 Dinners

Dinner is a great place to start to break out your culinary tricks. By this point, you're becoming more comfortable in the kitchen and perhaps a bit more adventurous. You're ready to branch out into cooking foods you might once have been afraid to attempt. Not to worry—while these foods may taste amazing (and even create some new Health Fix addictions!), they are also a snap to prepare.

Herbed Mustard Salmon

1½ pounds salmon fillet

1 teaspoon lemon juice

Pinch of salt

Pinch of ground black pepper

3 tablespoons Dijon mustard

½ cup chopped scallions

½ cup chopped parsley

½ cup chopped fresh dill

Preheat the oven to 350°F. Rinse the salmon and pat dry with paper towels. Place the salmon skin side down on a baking dish coated with cooking spray. Season the fish with the lemon juice, salt, and pepper. Spread the mustard over the top of the fish evenly. Spread the scallions, parsley, and dill on top of the mustard. Bake the salmon for 20 to 30 minutes, or until the fish is opaque.

Makes 4 servings

Per serving: 262 calories, 34 g protein, 4 g carbohydrates, 11 g total fat, 2 g saturated fat, 1 g fiber, 388 mg sodium

Broccoli with Garlic and Ginger

1 bunch broccoli (1 pound), washed and chopped into florets

2 teaspoons olive oil

2 cloves garlic, chopped

1 tablespoon minced fresh ginger

$\frac{1}{4}$ teaspoon salt

$\frac{1}{4}$ teaspoon ground black pepper

Cook the broccoli in a steam basket for 3 minutes, or until it is just beginning to soften. Remove from the heat. Heat the oil in a large skillet over medium-high heat. Add the garlic and ginger. Cook, stirring frequently, for 1 to 2 minutes. Add the broccoli to the skillet. Continue cooking, stirring frequently, for 3 to 5 minutes. Season the broccoli with the salt and pepper.

Makes 3 servings

Per serving: 73 calories, 4 g protein, 9 g carbohydrate, 3 g total fat, 0 g saturated fat, 3 g fiber, 237 mg sodium

Chicken Stir-Fry

1 large carrot, chopped

1 cup cauliflower florets

1 cup sugar snap peas

2 tablespoons reduced-sodium soy sauce

2 tablespoons rice wine vinegar

2 teaspoons cornstarch

1 teaspoon agave syrup

¼ teaspoon red pepper flakes

1 tablespoon sesame oil

2 cloves garlic, sliced

1 tablespoon minced fresh ginger

8 ounces shiitake or button mushrooms, sliced

1 medium red bell pepper, sliced

3 cups boneless skinless chicken breast (page 236), cut into strips

¼ cup sliced scallions

Fill a medium pot with salted water and bring to a boil. Add the carrot and cauliflower. After 1 minute, add the sugar snaps. Let the vegetables cook 1 more minute and strain. Rinse with cold water and set aside. In a small bowl, whisk together the soy sauce, vinegar, cornstarch, agave, and red-pepper flakes and set aside. In a large skillet or wok, heat the sesame oil over medium-high heat. Add the garlic and ginger. Cook for 1 to 2 minutes. Add the mushrooms and cook for another 2 to 3 minutes. Add the chicken, red bell pepper, and the blanched carrot, cauliflower, and sugar snaps. Pour the soy sauce mixture over the chicken and vegetables. Mix to evenly coat. Once everything is heated through, add the scallions and cook 1 more minute.

Makes 3 servings

Per serving: 374 calories, 48 g protein, 21 g carbohydrate, 10 g total fat, 2 g saturated fat, 6 g fiber, 581 mg sodium

Variation: Shrimp Stir-Fry: Decrease the soy sauce to 1 tablespoon and replace the chicken with 1 pound cooked shrimp.

Per serving: 299 calories, 35 g protein, 21 g carbohydrate, 8 g total fat, 1 g saturated fat, 6 g fiber, 359 mg sodium

Turkey Meat Loaf

1½ pounds lean ground turkey

2 large cloves garlic, minced

½ cup chopped onion

½ cup whole wheat, dried bread crumbs

⅓ cup fat-free milk

2 eggs, beaten

2 tablespoons parsley

1 tablespoon Worcestershire sauce

1 tablespoon Dijon mustard

1 tablespoon capers

½ teaspoon salt

½ teaspoon ground black pepper

Preheat the oven to 375°F. In a large bowl, combine the ground turkey, garlic, onion, bread crumbs, milk, eggs, parsley, Worcestershire sauce, mustard, capers, salt, and pepper. Coat a loaf pan with cooking spray. Put the meat mixture into the loaf pan and bake for 45 to 55 minutes, or until a thermometer inserted in the center registers 165°F and the meat is no longer pink.

Makes 6 servings

Per serving: 244 calories, 26 g protein, 10 g carbohydrates, 11 g total fat, 3 g saturated fat, 1 g fiber, 392 mg sodium

Variation: Substitute the ground turkey with 1½ pounds lean ground beef to make a traditional meat loaf.

Per serving: 276 calories, 27 g protein, 10 g carbohydrate, 13 g total fat, 5 g saturated fat, 1 g fiber, 401 mg sodium

Roasted Cauliflower

1 head cauliflower, washed, trimmed, and chopped into florets

2 cloves garlic, minced

2 tablespoons minced fresh ginger

1 tablespoon olive oil

$\frac{1}{4}$ teaspoon salt

$\frac{1}{4}$ teaspoon ground black pepper

1 teaspoon curry powder (optional)

$\frac{1}{2}$ teaspoon cardamom (optional)

$\frac{1}{4}$ teaspoon red pepper flakes (optional)

Preheat the oven to 400°F. In a medium bowl, combine the cauliflower, garlic, ginger, oil, salt, and pepper. Add the curry powder, cardamom, and red pepper flakes (if using). Toss well. Place in a baking pan or baking dish. Cover with foil. Roast in the oven for 20 minutes, or until the cauliflower is golden and soft.

Makes 4 servings

Per serving: 71 calories, 3 g protein, 8 g carbohydrate, 4 g total fat, 1 g saturated fat, 3 g fiber, 191 mg sodium

Green Beans with Roasted Garlic and Lemon

1 pound fresh green beans

2 large cloves garlic, roasted and chopped (see note)

2 teaspoons olive oil

$\frac{1}{4}$ teaspoon salt

$\frac{1}{4}$ teaspoon ground black pepper

2 tablespoons lemon juice

$\frac{1}{2}$ teaspoon grated lemon peel

$\frac{1}{4}$ cup roasted, sliced almonds (optional)

Wash and trim the green beans. Cook the green beans in a steam basket for 5 minutes, or until they are just beginning to soften. Remove from the heat. Heat the oil in a large skillet over medium-high heat. Add the roasted garlic. Cook, stirring frequently, for 1 minute. Add the green beans. Continue cooking, stirring frequently, for 5 minutes. Add the salt and pepper. Toss with the lemon juice and lemon peel. Garnish with the almonds (if using).

Makes 3 servings

Per serving: 79 calories, 3 g protein, 12 g carbohydrate, 3 g total fat, 0 g saturated fat, 4 g fiber, 206 mg sodium

Note: To roast garlic, preheat the oven to 350°F. Wrap peeled garlic cloves with a small sheet of foil. Roast for 20 to 25 minutes. The garlic should be soft and fragrant, but not burnt.

Roasted Pork Loin

1 teaspoon olive oil

1 clove garlic, minced

$\frac{1}{2}$ teaspoon salt

$\frac{1}{4}$ teaspoon ground black pepper

2–3 pounds pork loin

Preheat the oven to 350°F. Rub the oil, garlic, salt, and pepper into the pork loin. Place the pork loin in a roasting pan. Roast for 1½ to 2 hours, or until a thermometer inserted in the center registers 155°F and the juices run clear. Let the pork sit for 5 to 10 minutes prior to carving.

Makes 5–8 servings

Per serving: 335 calories, 52 g protein, 0 g carbohydrate, 13 g total fat, 4 g saturated fat, 0 g fiber, 187 mg sodium

Variations : Teriyaki Pork Loin: Replace the olive oil, garlic, salt, and pepper with Teriyaki Marinade (page 257). Marinate the loin for at least 15 minutes. Remove from the marinade before cooking.

Per serving: 331 calories, 52 g protein, 1 g carbohydrate, 12 g total fat, 4 g saturated fat, 0 g fiber, 160 mg sodium

Red Wine Marinated Pork Loin: Replace the olive oil, garlic, salt, and pepper with Red Wine Marinade (page 256). Marinate the pork loin in the Red Wine Marinade for at least 15 minutes. Remove from the marinade before cooking.

Per serving: 330 calories, 51 g protein, 0 g carbohydrate, 12 g total fat, 4 g saturated fat, 0 g fiber, 109 mg sodium

Stage 3 Dinners

I hope by this point, you've begun to invite others over to enjoy your gourmet meals! Don't be shy—show off both your newfound cooking skills and the fit, toned body under your apron. While everything about these dinners is a Healthy Fix, don't forget they were also created by Natalia Hancock, one of the nation's top culinary nutritionists at New York City's Rouge Tomate—so you're becoming a master by learning from a master herself!

Cioppino

1 tablespoon olive oil

4 cloves garlic, sliced

1 fennel bulb, sliced lengthwise

1 medium onion, sliced

1 sprig thyme

$\frac{1}{2}$ teaspoon ground black pepper

$\frac{1}{4}$ teaspoon red pepper flakes

1 can (28 ounces) whole tomatoes, chopped into 1" pieces
   (or 1$\frac{1}{2}$ fresh tomatoes, chopped)

2 cups clam juice

1 cup dry wine, red or white

$\frac{1}{2}$ cup water

1 bay leaf

1 pound white fish (see note), cut into 2" chunks

$\frac{1}{2}$ pound peeled and deveined shrimp

$\frac{1}{2}$ pound small bay scallops

$\frac{1}{2}$ pound cleaned and rinsed mussels or clams

$\frac{1}{2}$ cup chopped parsley

Heat the oil in a large skillet over medium-high heat. Add the garlic, fennel, onion, thyme, black pepper, and red pepper flakes. Cook, stirring frequently, for 4 to 5 minutes, or until soft. Add the tomatoes (with juice), clam juice, wine, water, and bay leaf. Cover the skillet and bring to a boil. Reduce the heat and simmer for 20 minutes. Add the seafood and stir to combine. Cook uncovered for 5 to 6 minutes, or until the seafood is just cooked through. Remove and discard the sprig of thyme and bay leaf. Garnish with the parsley.

Makes 4 servings

Per serving: 374 calories, 50 g protein, 25 g carbohydrates, 7 g total fat, 1 g saturated fat, 5 g fiber, 1361 mg sodium

Note: Any white fish can be used, such as halibut, cod, hake, and pollock.

Whole Grain Croutons

   4 slices or 4 ounces stale or whole grain toasted bread

   Olive oil cooking spray

   $1/2$ teaspoon paprika

   $1/4$ teaspoon salt

   $1/4$ teaspoon ground black pepper

Preheat the oven to 425°F. Slice the bread into $1/2''$ cubes. Lightly coat the bread cubes with the cooking spray. Toss with the paprika, salt, and pepper. Place on a baking sheet. Bake for 5 minutes, or until golden and crisp. The croutons can be stored in a resealable plastic bag for a week.

Makes 4 servings

Per serving: 75 calories, 4 g protein, 12 g carbohydrate, 1 g total fat, 0 g saturated fat, 2 g fiber, 280 mg sodium

Turkey Meatballs

2 tablespoons minced onion

1 small clove garlic, minced

1 pound lean ground turkey (see note)

1 egg, beaten

$\frac{1}{4}$ cup whole wheat bread crumbs

$\frac{1}{4}$ cup fat-free Greek yogurt

$\frac{1}{2}$ teaspoon salt

$\frac{1}{4}$ teaspoon ground black pepper

Preheat the oven to 375°F. Coat a small skillet with cooking spray and heat over medium-high heat. Add the onion and garlic. Cook, stirring frequently, for 1 minute. In a large bowl, combine the turkey, sautéed onion and garlic, egg, bread crumbs, yogurt, salt, and pepper. Mix well. Coat a baking sheet with cooking spray. Form the turkey mixture into 1$\frac{1}{2}$"-thick meatballs. Bake for 20 minutes, or until a thermometer inserted registers 170°F. Great when served with sautéed zucchini (page 233).

Makes 4 servings

Per serving: 223 calories, 26 g protein, 6 g carbohydrate, 10 g total fat, 3 g saturated fat, 0 g fiber, 432 mg sodium

Notes: Ground chicken or lean ground beef can also be used.

Stuffed Flounder

1½ pounds flounder or other white fish (4 small, thin fillets)

1 teaspoon olive oil

2 tablespoons lemon juice, divided

1 clove garlic, minced

1 tablespoon capers

2 tablespoons chopped dill

2 tablespoons chopped chives

2 tablespoons chopped parsley

¼ teaspoon ground black pepper

1 teaspoon paprika

Pinch of salt

Preheat the oven to 350°F. Lay out the flounder fillets flat side down on a clean, dry surface. Drizzle the fish with the olive oil and 1 tablespoon of the lemon juice. Spread the garlic, capers, dill, chives, and parsley evenly over the fillets. Season the fillets with the pepper. Roll each fillet starting with the smaller end. Coat an appropriately sized baking dish with cooking spray. Place each rolled filet in the dish. Season each filet with the remaining lemon juice, paprika, and salt. Bake for 30 to 35 minutes, or until the fish is opaque in the center.

Makes 4 servings

Per serving: 116 calories, 18 g protein, 1 g carbohydrate, 4 g total fat, 1 g saturated fat, 0 g fiber, 522 mg sodium

Lasagna

1 large zucchini, sliced lengthwise into 4 slices $\frac{1}{2}$" thick

$1\frac{1}{2}$ teaspoons salt, divided

$\frac{1}{2}$ teaspoon ground black pepper, divided

$\frac{1}{2}$ slice stale bread

2 tablespoons milk

1 teaspoon olive oil

1 small onion, chopped, divided

3 cloves garlic, minced, divided

$\frac{1}{2}$ pound ground turkey (see note)

10 ounces (1 package) button mushrooms, sliced

4–6 cups tomato sauce

1 cup reduced-fat or fat-free ricotta, divided

1 cup reduced-fat mozzarella, divided

Set the oven to broil. Spray the 4 zucchini slices with nonstick cooking spray on each side and season with $\frac{1}{2}$ teaspoon of the salt and $\frac{1}{4}$ teaspoon of the ground black pepper. Lay the zucchini flat on a baking sheet. Broil on each side for 1 to 2 minutes, or until the slices are lightly golden brown. Set the browned zucchini aside. Soak the bread in milk and set aside. Heat the olive oil in a large skillet over medium-high heat. Cook half of the onion and garlic for 1 to 2 minutes, stirring frequently. Add the ground turkey and start browning, being careful not to break up the turkey too much. Add another $\frac{1}{2}$ teaspoon of the salt and the remaining ground black pepper. Squeeze the milk from the bread into the turkey and mix well. The milk will keep leaner ground meats from drying out. Discard the bread. Once the turkey is mostly browned, remove it from the skillet and set aside. Return the skillet to the burner and add the sliced mushrooms and the remaining onion and garlic. Cook for 5 minutes, then add the remaining salt. Cook another few minutes until any moisture is cooked off. Set aside.

To assemble the lasagna: Preheat the oven to 375°F. Place $\frac{1}{4}$ cup of the tomato sauce in the bottom of an ovenproof 9" x 9" baking dish. Lay 2 of the broiled zucchini slices in the bottom of the dish. Take $\frac{1}{4}$ cup of ricotta cheese and spread it over the broiled zucchini slices. Sprinkle each slice with 1 tablespoon of the mozzarella. Layer all of the turkey over the zucchini and cheese, then cover with 2 cups of the sauce. Spread the remaining ricotta over the last 2 slices of zucchini and layer them with 2 tablespoons of the mozzarella. Add the sautéed mushrooms over the top of the cheese. Cover the lasagna with the remaining sauce and then sprinkle the remaining cheese over the top. Bake for 35 to 45 minutes to an hour, until cheese is bubbly.

Makes 4 servings

Per serving: 416 calories, 32 g protein, 27 g carbohydrate, 21 g total fat, 8 g saturated fat, 6 g fiber, 1596 mg sodium

Note: TVP, chicken, or beef can be substituted for the turkey.

Roasted Asparagus

1 pound asparagus (1 bunch)

2 cloves garlic, chopped

1 tablespoon olive oil

1 tablespoon lemon juice

¼ teaspoon salt

¼ teaspoon ground black pepper

Preheat the oven to 400°F. Wash and trim the asparagus, removing the woody bottoms (the bottom 1"–2"). In a baking dish, toss the asparagus, garlic, and olive oil. Roast in the oven for 15 to 20 minutes, depending on the thickness of the asparagus. Season the asparagus with the lemon juice, salt, and pepper prior to serving.

Makes 3 servings

Per serving: 69 calories, 3 g protein, 6 g carbohydrates, 5 g total fat, 1 g saturated fat, 3 g fiber, 199 mg sodium

Shepherd's Pie

Meat

2 teaspoons olive oil

1 pound grass-fed ground beef

2 large cloves garlic, minced

2 cups sliced mushrooms

$\frac{1}{2}$ cup chopped onion

$\frac{1}{4}$ cup chopped celery

$\frac{1}{4}$ cup grated carrot (1 small carrot)

$\frac{1}{4}$ teaspoon salt

$\frac{1}{4}$ teaspoon ground black pepper

Smashed Potatoes

1 pound thin-skinned potatoes (new, Yukon, or Red Bliss), washed
and chopped into 1" pieces, skin on

1 teaspoon salt

2 cloves roasted garlic (see note on page 301)

$\frac{3}{4}$–1 cup fat-free milk

2 teaspoons olive oil

$\frac{1}{4}$ teaspoon ground black pepper

1–1$\frac{1}{2}$ cups cream-style corn

For the meat: Heat the oil in a large skillet over medium-high heat. Add the ground beef, garlic, mushrooms, onion, celery, carrot, salt, and pepper. Cook, stirring frequently, for 5 minutes, or until the meat browns.

For the smashed potatoes: Preheat the oven to 375°F. In a medium pot, add the potatoes and cover with cold water. Add the salt. Bring to a boil, reduce the heat, and simmer for 15 minutes, or until the potatoes are tender. Strain the potatoes and mash with the roasted garlic, milk, oil, and pepper. In an ovenproof 9" x 9" baking dish, layer the meat mixture. Then add the smashed potatoes over the meat. Top with the corn. Bake 20 to 30 minutes, or until heated all the way through.

Makes 4 servings

Per serving: 421 calories, 28 g protein, 36 g carbohydrates, 20 g total fat, 7 g saturated fat, 5 g fiber, 344 mg sodium

Snacks

Some of these snacks might seem a bit oddball at first, but give them a try. Kale chips are a supernutritious stand-in for potato chips or crackers—and so delicious! Most can be prepared ahead of time and taken along to give you energy and head off any False Fix urges on the go.

Deviled Eggs

6 eggs (see note)

¼ cup fat-free Greek yogurt

1 tablespoon capers

1 tablespoon minced celery

1 tablespoon chopped chives

1 tablespoon chopped parsley

1 teaspoon Dijon mustard

¼ teaspoon ground black pepper

Dash of Tabasco sauce

¼ teaspoon smoked paprika

12 small sprigs dill

In a large pot, place the eggs and cover with cold water. Bring to a boil, turn off the heat, and cover. Let the eggs sit in the hot water covered for 10 minutes. Remove and run the eggs under cold water. When the eggs are cool enough to handle, remove the shells. Carefully halve the eggs lengthwise. Remove the yolks and place the yolks in a medium bowl. Add the yogurt, capers, celery, chives, parsley, mustard, pepper, and Tabasco. Mix well. Fill each halved egg with the yolk mixture. Garnish with the smoked paprika and sprigs of dill.

Makes 6 servings

Per serving: 85 calories, 7 g protein, 1 g carbohydrate, 5 g total fat, 2 g saturated fat, 0 g fiber, 129 mg sodium

Note: This recipe works best when the eggs are still warm.

Kale Chips

1 bunch of kale, washed, cut into 2" pieces with ribs removed
  (about 3 cups)
1 tablespoon olive oil
½ teaspoon salt

Preheat the oven to 325°F. Toss the kale with the olive oil and salt. Place on a baking sheet. Bake for 10 to 15 minutes, mixing once halfway through. The kale should be crispy but not browned.

Makes 4 servings

Per serving: 51 calories, 1 g protein, 4 g carbohydrate, 4 g total fat, 1 g saturated fat, 1 g fiber, 330 mg sodium

Chia Pudding

1½ cups fat-free plain Greek yogurt
1 cup vanilla soy milk
¼ cup cherry juice (optional)
2 tablespoons chia seeds
2 tablespoons dried cherries (see note)
¼ teaspoon ground cinnamon (optional)

In a medium bowl, combine the yogurt, soy milk, cherry juice (if using), chia seeds, dried cherries, and cinnamon (if using). Mix well. Cover and refrigerate for at least 1 hour.

Makes 2 servings

Per serving: 219 calories, 20 g protein, 23 g carbohydrate, 5 g total fat, 1 g saturated fat, 5 g fiber, 99 mg sodium

Note: Any other dried fruit can be substituted for the cherries.

Tzatziki Sauce

1 small Persian or Kirby cucumber, finely chopped

1 teaspoon salt

1 cup fat-free Greek yogurt

1 clove garlic, roasted and minced (see note)

1 tablespoon chopped fresh dill

1 tablespoon chopped fresh parsley

1 teaspoon grated lemon peel

1 teaspoon lemon juice

¼ teaspoon black pepper

Place the chopped cucumber into a strainer and sprinkle the salt over it. The salt will draw the moisture out of the cucumber. Let it sit for at least 15 minutes in the strainer, and then dab the cucumber with a paper towel to remove excess moisture. In a bowl, combine the cucumber with the yogurt, roasted garlic, dill, parsley, lemon peel, lemon juice, and pepper. Let it sit for 10 minutes before serving.

Makes 4 servings (1 cup)

Per serving: 41 calories, 5 g protein, 5 g carbohydrate, 0 g total fat, 0 g saturated fat, 0 g fiber, 313 mg sodium

Note: Preheat the oven to 350°F. Wrap peeled garlic cloves with a small sheet of foil. Roast for 20 to 25 minutes. The garlic should be soft and fragrant, but not burnt.

Fresh Melon Granita

1 honeydew melon, seeded and diced

2 tablespoons lime juice

1 tablespoon grated lime peel

In a large bowl, puree the melon. Add the lime juice and peel. Freeze in a shallow dish for 45 minutes to an hour. The melon should be not fully frozen. Shave with spoon and serve. Garnish with a fresh lime.

Makes 6 servings

Per serving: 79 calories, 1 g protein, 20 g carbohydrate, 0 g total fat, 0 g saturated fat, 2 g fiber, 39 mg sodium

Hummus

1 can (15 ounces) chickpeas, rinsed and drained

¼ cup water

3 tablespoons lemon juice

1 clove garlic, minced

½ teaspoon ground cumin

½ teaspoon salt

Pinch of ground red pepper

3 tablespoons tahini

1 tablespoon olive oil

In a food processor, combine the chickpeas, water, lemon juice, garlic, cumin, salt, and pepper. Process for 30 seconds. Scrape down the sides of the bowl and process for another 30 seconds. Whisk the tahini and olive oil in a small bowl. With the processor running, stream the oil and tahini mixture into the bowl. Process for another 15 to 30 seconds until the hummus is smooth.

Makes 6 servings (1½ cups)

Per serving: 183 calories, 8 g protein, 22 g carbohydrate, 8 g total fat, 1 g saturated fat, 6 g fiber, 208 mg sodium

Variation: Add roasted garlic or roasted red bell peppers for a twist on the flavor.

Berry Yogurt Frozen Ice Pops

1–2 cups frozen mixed berries, thawed

½ cup fat-free Greek yogurt

½ cup fat-free or 1% milk

In a large bowl, combine the berries, yogurt, and milk. With a stick blender, process the mixture until smooth. Pour into ice pop molds and freeze as directed by the manufacturer. Depending on the size and number of your molds, you may need to adjust the quantities. Any leftover mixture can be frozen for use in smoothies.

Makes 4

Per serving: 48 calories, 4 g protein, 9 g carbohydrate, 0 g total fat, 0 g saturated fat, 2 g fiber, 21 mg sodium

Appendix A

The Yale Food Addiction Scale

THIS IS THE LONG VERSION (SEE PAGE 22 FOR THE SHORT version) of the scientifically validated Yale Food Addiction Scale.[1] It gives you an accurate gauge of the likelihood that you are addicted to certain foods. Please be completely honest with yourself—taking this test will help you gauge the extent to which False Fixes have a grip on you.

IN THE PAST 12 MONTHS:	Never	Once a month	2–4 times a month	2–3 times a week	4 or more times a week or daily
1. I find that when I start eating certain foods, I end up eating much more than planned.	0	1	2	3	4
2. I find myself continuing to consume certain foods even though I am no longer hungry.	0	1	2	3	4
3. I eat to the point where I feel physically ill.	0	1	2	3	4
4. Not eating certain types of food or cutting down on certain types of food is something I worry about.	0	1	2	3	4
5. I spend a lot of time feeling sluggish or fatigued from overeating.	0	1	2	3	4
6. I find myself constantly eating certain foods throughout the day.	0	1	2	3	4
7. I find that when certain foods are not available, I will go out of my way to obtain them. For example, I will drive to the store to purchase certain foods even though I have other options available to me at home.	0	1	2	3	4

IN THE PAST 12 MONTHS:	Never	Once a month	2–4 times a month	2–3 times a week	4 or more times a week or daily
8. There have been times when I consumed certain foods so often or in such large quantities that I started to eat food instead of working, spending time with my family or friends, or engaging in other important activities or recreational activities I enjoy.	0	1	2	3	4
9. There have been times when I consumed certain foods so often or in such large quantities that I spent time dealing with negative feelings from overeating instead of working, spending time with my family or friends, or engaging in other important activities or recreational activities I enjoy.	0	1	2	3	4

IN THE PAST 12 MONTHS:	Never	Once a month	2–4 times a month	2–3 times a week	4 or more times a week or daily
10. There have been times when I avoided professional or social situations where certain foods were available, because I was afraid I would overeat.	0	1	2	3	4
11. There have been times when I avoided professional or social situations because I was not able to consume certain foods there.	0	1	2	3	4
12. I have had withdrawal symptoms such as agitation, anxiety, or other physical symptoms when I cut down or stopped eating certain foods. (Please do NOT include withdrawal symptoms caused by cutting down on caffeinated beverages such as soda pop, coffee, tea, energy drinks, etc.)	0	1	2	3	4

IN THE PAST 12 MONTHS:	Never	Once a month	2–4 times a month	2–3 times a week	4 or more times a week or daily
13. I have consumed certain foods to prevent feelings of anxiety, agitation, or other physical symptoms that were developing. (Please do NOT include consumption of caffeinated beverages such as soda pop, coffee, tea, energy drinks, etc.)	0	1	2	3	4
14. I have found that I have elevated desire for or urges to consume certain foods when I cut down or stop eating them.	0	1	2	3	4
15. My behavior with respect to food and eating causes significant distress.	0	1	2	3	4
16. I experience significant problems in my ability to function effectively (daily routine, job/school, social activities, family activities, health difficulties) because of food and eating.	0	1	2	3	4

IN THE PAST 12 MONTHS (Y=1; N=0):

17. My food consumption has caused significant psychological problems such as depression, anxiety, self-loathing, or guilt. (Y/N)

18. My food consumption has caused significant physical problems or made a physical problem worse. (Y/N)

19. I kept consuming the same types of food or the same amount of food even though I was having emotional and/or physical problems. (Y/N)

20. Over time, I have found that I need to eat more and more to get the feeling I want, such as reduced negative emotions or increased pleasure. (Y/N)

21. I have found that eating the same amount of food does not reduce my negative emotions or increase pleasurable feelings the way it used to. (Y/N)

22. I want to cut down or stop eating certain kinds of food. (Y/N)

23. I have tried to cut down or stop eating certain kinds of food.

24. I have been successful at cutting down or not eating these kinds of food. (Y/N)

How many times in the past year did you try to cut down or stop eating certain foods altogether?

1 time

2 times

3 times

4 times

5 or more times

Please circle ALL of the following foods you have problems with:

Ice cream	Candy	Crackers	Bacon
Chocolate	White bread	Chips	Hamburgers
Apples	Rolls	Pretzels	Cheeseburgers
Doughnuts	Lettuce	French fries	Pizza
Broccoli	Pasta	Carrots	Soda pop
Cookies	Strawberries	Steak	None of the
Cake	Rice	Bananas	above

If you've scored above a 1 on any of the questions above, you are on the spectrum of food addiction. The list below will help you ascertain your biggest warning flags for trouble areas.

1. Substance taken in larger amount and for longer period than intended.
   Questions #1, #2, #3

2. Persistent desire or repeated unsuccessful attempt to quit.
   Questions #4, #22, # 24, #25

3. Much time/activity to obtain, use, recover.
   Questions #5, #6, #7

4. Important social, occupational, or recreational activities given up or reduced.
   Questions #8, #9, #10, #11

5. Use continues despite knowledge of adverse consequences (e.g., failure to fulfill role obligation, use when physically hazardous).
   Question #19

6. Tolerance (marked increase in amount; marked decrease in effect).
   Questions #20, #21

7. Characteristic withdrawal symptoms; substance taken to relieve withdrawal.
   Questions #12, #13, #14

8. Use causes clinically significant impairment.
   Questions #15, #16

Appendix B

Mind-Mouth-Muscle Daily Journal		
NAME:		**DATE:**
Mind	**Muscle**	**Mouth**
Today I will:	**Today I will:**	**Today I will:**
_____	_____	_____
_____	_____	_____
		_____
Video/Write: _____		Breakfast:
√ Meditation _____		
		Snack:
		Lunch:
		Snack:
		Dinner:
√ Meditation _____		

Appendix C

The Three Pillars
of the Hunger Fix

COMMITTING TO THE HUNGER FIX MEANS SETTING A positive intention around each of the three pillars of the program—the Three M's. Until you have your own mantra in place, you can use these affirmations as a place to start your Hunger Fix program.

Mind

I am powerful and I can control my mental and physical addictions to food. I commit to the regular practice of:

- Engaging in prayer and/or meditation
- Expressing gratitude for the blessings in my life
- Sustaining powerful and passionate meaning in my life
- Achieving joy through my achievements and giving to others
- Showing patience and persistence with my recovery process
- Seeking support when I need it
- Eliminating any persons, places, or things in my life that do not support my recovery
- Adapting and adjusting to life's stresses without self-destruction

- Being vigilant about making the best lifestyle choices
- Having faith that through courage, fortitude, honesty, and self-determination, I will achieve a lifelong recovery from food addiction

Mouth

I will choose those foods that will nourish me with life-giving nutrients. I commit to the regular practice of:

- Being abstinent of those foods and beverages that trigger my food addiction
- Selecting nonaddictive vegetables, fruits, whole grains, and lean proteins to provide me with the minerals, vitamins, and fiber I need to fuel my life's journey
- Being mindful of portions
- Eating delicious balanced meals and snacks every 3 or 4 hours
- Cooking as many meals and snacks as I can

Muscle

I acknowledge that my mind and body are one, and that by dealing with my mental weight I will be able to remove excess physical weight. I commit to the regular practice of:

- Engaging in some form of cardio activity for at least 30 minutes accrued five times per week
- Having fun and being joyful: participate in dance, play, walk, run, hike, bike, do sports
- Going inward with walking meditation, yoga, martial arts
- Getting strong through twice-a-week strength training
- Using my physical and mental power to help others

t), everyone will be tracking progress with their Clothes-O-Meter through-
Detox and beyond. The Clothes-O-Meter process is simple and fosters a new
healthy mind-body awareness—and hey, you have to wear clothes, so you'll
noticing the changes anyway.

Once you hit the beginning of Stage 2, however, I strongly suggest taking a
more objective measures so you can start to track your body's changes as you
progress from Detox through Recovery—because the changes will be significant.
And don't forget: Achievement is a massive dopamine booster and a natural high!
Watching the numbers fall while your body sheds addictive fat and gets leaner,
stronger, and more energetic will be a tremendous double-dip Healthy Fix.

Again, these body measurements are optional for day 1 of Detox but highly
recommended for day 1 of Stage 2. Measure and then write down your numbers
in the "Document Your Body Rewards" chart opposite.

Body quantity. Know your weight: Wake up in the morning and write
down your first weight. After visiting the bathroom, hop on your scale.

Body quality. Know your body fat percentage: After you have recorded
your body weight, we'll need a body fat percentage. Many home scales
have this feature built in. If you'd like a more accurate gauge, ask your
doctor (or a certified fitness professional at the gym) to measure your
body fat. In Stage 2, you'll start paying attention to this as an indicator of
how much fat and muscle you have, or your body composition. The more
fit and compact you are, the smaller and more powerful your body is.

Body size. This is where you use your Clothes-O-Meter. In addition, I
highly recommend that you whip out a tape measure and do a few day 1
recordings: the girth across your belly button and your lower abdominal
pooch (the largest part of your belly). Beyond that, you have several
additional options: midthigh, mid–upper arm, chest across your breasts,
chest below your breasts. These numbers will help you understand your
amazing achievements as you progress.

Note: These objective measures are also an antidote against the "buts"—
"Yeah, I'm down a size *but* I have *so* far to go." That's the negative inner addict
speaking. We shall have none of that! Instead, it's all about the "ands"—"Yes,
I'm down a size *and* I can't believe I've dropped 12 inches of fat from my body.
And I'm keepin' on track for more!" That's the voice of empowerment. We'll
revisit these measurements at the start of Stage 2 and Stage 3.

Appendix D

The Hunger Fix
Quick Shopping List

I F YOU'RE STARTING OUT ON THE PROGRAM, IT HELPS to stock
your larder with the raw materials for your successful Hunger Fix lifestyle.
Use this list to get your kitchen in order. But I know that buying all of this
at one time would be quite a financial hit to most food budgets! So to make this
shopping the most economically feasible, start with the freshest ingredients, and
add one of the condiments and seasonings to your shopping list every week.

Condiments and Seasonings

Condiments: mustard, hot sauce
(chipotle and regular), soy sauce,
Worcestershire sauce

Herbs, fresh or dried: dill, parsley,
cilantro, basil, oregano, chives,
scallions

Oils, cooking: olive, canola, peanut,
sesame

Oils, drizzling: extra-virgin olive, nut
oils; cold pressed, infused

Spices: cayenne, chili powder, cumin,
cinnamon, curry, smoked paprika,

dry mustard, nutmeg, red pepper
flakes, ginger, turmeric, celery seed,
cloves

Sweeteners (to be used sparingly):
Brown sugar, granulated sugar, agave
syrup, Stevia in the Raw, honey

Stock: chicken, fish, beef, or
vegetable, low-sodium canned (or,
ideally, made fresh!)

Vinegar: balsamic, rice wine, red
wine, sherry, distilled and cider
vinegar

Grains

Barley	Quinoa
Brown rice	Stone-ground oats
Bulgur	Wasa whole grain crackers
High-fiber cereal	Wheat berries
Oat bran	Wheat germ
Old-fashioned oats	Whole wheat bread crumbs
Popcorn kernels	Whole wheat flour

Nuts, Seeds, and Legumes

Legumes, canned: kidney beans, chickpeas, pinto beans, black beans, white beans (ones with no BPA)

Legumes, dried: split peas, lentils, chickpeas, black-eyed peas

Nut butters: peanut, almond, cashew

Nuts: almonds, peanuts, walnuts, hazelnuts, pecans, cashews, Brazil nuts

Seeds: Sesame, chia, pumpkin, flaxseed

Dairy and Plant Milks

Cottage cheese (low-fat)

Milk: low-fat or fat-free dairy, soy milk, almond milk

Protein powders: egg, whey, or soy

ricotta cheese

Yogurt: fat-free Greek

Meat, Fish, and Eggs

Beef, lean

Chicken: whole, legs, breast, ground

Eggs

Fish, canned: tuna, salmon, sardines, kipper snacks (herring)

Fish, fresh: whatever kinds, whenever possible

Pork, loin

Produce

Carrots

Celery

Edamame, frozen

Fruit, dried: prunes, raisins, apple rings, apricots, figs

Fruit, fresh: any in season

Fruit, frozen: strawberries, blueberries, raspberries, blackberries, mango

Garlic

Lemons

Onions

Peas, frozen

Appendix E

Document Your Rewards

(or n
out
and
be

fev
pr
A
w
s

YOU'LL NOTICE THAT FOR DETOX AND ALL OF THE don't talk too much about body "goals." Instead, I want you your achievements are not just goals and objectives but real to yourself. You're gifting yourself with a healthier, stronger, more You're wrapping your newly powerful PFC with a red ribbon and pres to yourself while you relish the newly honed control you feel as you fa temptation and challenge to your willpower. After all, I've been promisin you'd be surrounded with a cloud of reward throughout Detox. What bette to do that then to reframe goals as self-rewards?

We read about the Clothes-O-Meter in Chapter 5. I chose this metric Detox so that you devote your precious mental energies to the work of abstai ing from the False Fixes and not to stress out about scale hopping and hourl body-weight changes. That kind of obsessive behavior just fuels your inner addict. Trust me, if you're following the Mind-Mouth-Muscle template, you'll be dropping body fat and overall body size. You don't need a lump of metal to confirm what your new mind-body association is already telling you.

However, many people like to add a few more objective measures to their program, and that's fine. For Stage 1, these measures are optional; at Stage 2, these are more important. Do what feels right to you. If you'd rather get yourself through Detox without stressing about numbers, that's great. If you'd rather get a baseline of numbers quantifying your Detox start, that's perfectly fine as well. Whether you're obtaining weight, body fat percentage, and tape measurements

Document Your Body Rewards

	Start of Stage 1	Start of Stage 2	Stage 2 Target	80% of Stage 2 Target	Length of Time Maintained	Start of Stage 3
Body Quantity (Weight)						
Body Quality (Body Fat Percentage)						
Body Size (Clothes-O-Meter)						
Body Size (Waist Measurement)						
Body Size (Lower Abs Measurement)						
Body Size (_____ Measurement)						
Body Size (_____ Measurement)						
Body Size (_____ Measurement)						

What Should My Goals Be?

Keep it simple. There is no magic body-weight number where you suddenly experience Nirvana. Instead, shoot for a healthy body-weight range and then just approximate your target. Log on to WebMD's free Food and Fitness Planner (www.webmd.com/diet/food-fitness-planner/default.htm) and set a goal. If you're a 5-foot-3 woman who weighs 250 pounds, clearly you want to head south of 200 for sure. How far south? That's the $60,000 question. Instead of tormenting yourself over numbers, here is another measurement option you can make:

Body weight. Have a look at the "normal" ranges, remembering that there is rarely an age factor assigned to these ranges. Then take the larger number in the range, add my Peeke Padding of 5 more pounds for every 25 pounds you need to drop, and use that as the ultimate goal.

For instance, the 5-foot-3 woman's "normal" weight range is 104 to 141 pounds.

> Take 141 and add 5 pounds for every 25-pound segment
> (250—141 = about four 25-pound segments):
> 4 segments x 5 pounds = 20 pounds of padding.

Therefore, 141 + 20 = about 160 pounds body-weight goal. This woman's reward/goal is to remove 90 pounds. If she sheds 80 percent of the 90 pounds (72 pounds) and maintains that loss for 6 months, she'll be able to transition to Stage 3. Once she has hit her 80 percent goal, she can either maintain this achievement for whatever length of time she desires or at some point can continue to shed more weight.

Body quality. It's so important for you to remember that the real goal is to improve the quality of your body—your body composition. Your weight alone is just one metric used to describe the quality of your body. Body fat percentage helps you appreciate how much excess body fat you're shedding as you strengthen and tone your muscles. You'll see that body fat percentages change slowly, as they are indicators of lots of changes going on inside you. These percentages let us know how much fat and muscle you have (along with bone, which is more of a constant). As you drop fat, so long as you're physically active, you'll be able to hold on to most of your muscle mass. For that matter, you'll build more as well. *Your body fat percentage drops as you shed excess body fat while also either maintaining or building your muscle mass.* If you try to drop weight without being active, then you'll lose precious muscle mass. Research shows that in a typical "diet" where people are not exercising, over 25 percent of the weight dropped is actually muscle. You want to avoid this. Also, your body fat percentage is an indicator of your physical activity. If you're active, your body fat will fall nicely. If you're inactive, even if your weight is dropping, your body fat won't, since your muscle is dropping right along with your body fat. So we know if you're cheatin' and not staying active by monitoring your body fat percentage.

If you want to concentrate more on the quality, not just the quantity, of your body weight, then you can simply follow your body fat percentages. Here's a quickie normal range guide for average people (including nonelite athletes):

Age-Adjusted Body Fat Percentage Recommendations

Women

Age	Underfat	Healthy Range	Overweight	Obese
20–40 yrs	Under 21%	21–33%	33–39%	Over 39%
41–60 yrs	Under 23%	23–35%	35–40%	Over 40%
61–79 yrs	Under 24%	24–36%	36–42%	Over 42%

Men

Age	Underfat	Healthy Range	Overweight	Obese
20–40 yrs	Under 8%	8–19%	19–25%	Over 25%
41–60 yrs	Under 11%	11–22%	22–27%	Over 27%
61–79 yrs	Under 13%	13–25%	25–30%	Over 30%

SOURCE: D. Gallagher et al., "Healthy Percentage Body Fat Ranges: An Approach for Developing Guidelines Based on Body Mass Index," *American Journal of Clinical Nutrition* 72, no. 3 (September 2000):694–701.

Body size. Know your Clothes-O-Meter fit: Believe it or not, I have men and women in my practice who have never stepped on a scale and who don't know their body fat percentage; they simply use their clothing size as an indicator of their healthy weight and body composition. And they've done just fine. They've used their Clothes-O-Meters to carefully monitor size as they remove excess weight until they reach a place where they feel healthy and fit. Hey, if this is the only option that you feel comfortable with for tracking your progress, then so be it.

Appendix F

The Three M's: Resources

Mind: Learn How to Meditate

Whether you choose Transcendental Meditation, mindfulness, or any other type of meditation, you will reap tremendous Healthy Fix benefits. Just explore and you'll find the kind that works for you.

Benson-Henry Institute for Mind Body Medicine: www.massgeneral.org/bhi

Transcendence: Healing and Transformation Through Transcendental Meditation by Norman E. Rosenthal, MD (Viking, 2011)

Transcendental Meditation: www.tm.org; www.davidlynchfoundation.org

University of Massachusetts Center for Mindfulness: www.umassmed.edu/cfm/tny/index.aspx

Walking meditation: http://awakenedmind.net/walking-meditation-a-simple-guide

Zen meditation: www.mro.org/zmm/teachings/meditation.php

Mouth: Track Your Progress, Get Support, and Learn More About Nutrition

The more you learn about Healthy Fix foods, the more you'll want to know! Relish the world of fresh, whole, nutritious foods, and keep those dopamine levels high by continuing to challenge yourself in the kitchen.

Center for Science in the Public Interest: www.cspinet.org

Overeaters Anonymous: www.oa.org

Rouge Tomate: www.rougetomatenyc.com

SPE (Sanitas Per Escam or Health Through Nutrition): www.SPEcertified.com

WebMD Food and Fitness Planner: www.webmd.com/diet/food-fitness-planner/default.htm; also available as iPhone and iPad apps

Why Calories Count: From Science to Politics by Marion Nestle and Malden Nesheim (University of California Press, 2012)

DR. PEEKE'S EARLIER BOOKS

Fight Fat After Forty (Viking, 2000)

Body-for-Life for Women (Rodale, 2005)

Fit to Live (Rodale, 2007)

RESOURCES ON FOOD ADDICTION FOR HEALTH PROFESSIONALS

Epigenetics: http://the-scientist.com/2011/03/01/epigenetics—a-primer-2/

Food and Addiction, edited by Kelly Brownell and Art Gold (Oxford Press, 2012)

National Institute of Drug Abuse (NIDA): www.drugabuse.gov

Muscle: Move That Body

Once you start moving your body, you realize there is no end to the number of people and places waiting to help you. Here are a few of my favorites to help get beginners (or those of you who've been out of the game for a while) rehooked on the Healthy Fix of exercise.

- **Anytime Fitness.** This offers 24-hour locations and a great online Anytime Health program with healthy lifestyle content, all in an affordable program. www.anytimefitness.com

- **Community centers.** With affordable neighborhood locations, many towns' community centers feature dance classes, swimming lessons, running clubs, and other group fitness activities. These are especially helpful for folks with young kids or for seniors who are looking for more social time. Search online for a community center in your area.

- **Curves.** Gender specific, low stress, and no judgment—what could be better? Curves' new lifestyle program includes support for all your Mind and Mouth changes, too. Their program is affordable and has many locations to keep things convenient. (Bonus: Many Curves locations also feature Zumba!) www.curves.com

- **Equinox.** These gyms are higher end, with more bells and whistles including a spa, pool, and the latest cutting-edge exercise classes. www.equinox.com

- **Pilates.** The core is king—and Pilates gives you an integrated system to strengthen the core muscles using a floor mat or the Pilates reformer. Easy to do at home, Pilates is flexible enough so that you can follow DVDs or take classes. I can't stress this point enough: It is so important to maintain a powerful core and, as a result, a strong back and optimal posture. Search online for a Pilates studio in your area.

- **YMCA.** For many decades, the Y has offered great, affordable programs in good locations. One thing many parents really appreciate is that their kids can take classes or hang out in the childcare center while Mom and Dad use the gym or take their own fitness classes. Use of the pool on family nights is another huge perk of many YMCAs nationwide. www.ymca.net

- **Yoga.** There are many forms of yoga to choose from. Check out www.yogafit.com to learn more. Restorative is gentle and effective, especially for people with arthritis and physical disabilities. Bikram is the hot yoga option for folks who want to experience a real physical challenge with kindred spirits. Check out options at your gym or community center, via online apps, or through DVDs. Gaiam.com is a great source of the latest yoga offerings.

- **Zumba.** Through DVDs or classes in locations ranging from health clubs to church halls, you can experience a very different "tribe" or culture—dance, hot music, and group movement, all with specialized toning classes with strength training. There's also Zumba Gold, which is more gentle for folks "of a certain age." www.zumba.com

BEST APPS FOR THE HUNGER FIX LIFESTYLE

My patients are always asking for tools to help them resist False Fixes and make good choices on the go. Here are some of the most healthy apps, including those selected in the most recent US Surgeon General's Healthy Apps Challenge.[1]

Physical Activity

Lose It! in the category of fitness/physical activity

Fit Friendzy

MapMyFitness

iMuscle

RunKeeper

Livestrong

Family Fitness and Health

Max's Plate

Short Sequence: Kids' Yoga Journey

Nutrition/Healthy Eating

WebMD Food and Fitness Planner

GoodGuide

Fooducate

Integrative Health

Healthy Habits

Appendix G

Find Your Healthy Fix Voice

WHEN YOU STRUGGLE WITH FOOD ADDICTION, ONE OF your False Fixes is the negative, disempowering way you speak to yourself. Part of the Hunger Fix journey is learning to counter the False Fix lies you hear in your head and to adopt the Healthy Fix voice instead. Each stage has its own unique challenges; when you hear that False Fix lie coming into your head, counter it with a few of these powerful statements from your new Healthy Fix voice.

Stage 1 : Detox

False Fix Lie	Healthy Fix Voice
It's *just* a cookie, for crying out loud.	No way. This makes me lose control.
You'll never last. You never do.	I will make it. I'm saving my own life.
I have so far to go. I'll never make it.	I'm taking one day at a time. I'll make it.
This is so hard.	I accept the work I must do to change.
I'm a loser and I'll never hit my goal.	I'm a winner because I'm working it now.

Stage 2 : Beginner Recovery

False Fix Lie	Healthy Fix Voice
Life stress is just too much. I need food.	I can adapt and adjust to life's stresses.
People keep shoving food at me.	I'll stand firm with my choices.
I keep forgetting to eat/exercise.	If I fail to plan, I plan to fail.
This is so slow! I'll never get there.	Patience is the key to my success.
I'm not doing this perfectly.	Progress, not perfection, is my goal.
I slipped up and feel so bad.	I'll regroup and learn from each slip.
It's hard to focus and stay on track.	I am meditating and am mentally strong.

Stage 3 : Master Recovery

False Fix Lie	Healthy Fix Voice
You can eat anything now— you're thin!	I am fit, vigilant, and in recovery for life.
Can I really do this for a lifetime?	I believe in myself and lifelong recovery.
I'm afraid of relapsing.	Every day I will practice my vigilance.
I sometimes feel alone.	I have created a strong support system.
Can I really push myself more?	I'm embracing challenges with passion.

Notes

INTRODUCTION

1 A. Rayno, "When It Comes to Paychecks, Body Size Matters," *Washington Post,* January 20, 2011.

2 T. A. Judge and D. M. Cable, "When It Comes to Pay, Do the Thin Win? The Effect of Weight on Pay for Men and Women," *Journal of Applied Psychology* 96, no. 1 (January 2011):95–112. Published electronically September 20, 2010.

CHAPTER 1

1 http://forums.webmd.com/3/diet-exchange/forum/2500/27#27.

2 G. J. Wang, N. D. Volkow, et al., "Brain Dopamine and Obesity," *Lancet* 357, no. 9253 (February 3, 2001):354–57.

3 N. D. Volkow, " 'Nonhedonic' Food Motivation in Humans Involves Dopamine in the Dorsal Striatum and Methylphenidate Amplifies This Effect," *Synapse* 44, no. 3 (June 1, 2002):175–80.

4 A. Gearhardt et al., "Neural Correlates of Food Addiction," *Archives of General Psychiatry* 68, no. 8 (August 2011):808–16. Published electronically April 4, 2011.

5 N. D. Volkow, "Inverse Association Between BMI and Prefrontal Metabolic Activity in Healthy Adults," *Obesity* 17, no. 1 (2008), 60–65. doi:10.1038/oby.2008.469.

6 P. Johnson and P. J. Kenny, "Dopamine D2 Receptors in Addiction-Like Reward Dysfunction and Compulsive Eating in Obese Rats," *Nature Neuroscience* 13, no. 5 (2010):635–41.

7 M. M. Finucane et al., "National, Regional, and Global Trends in Body-Mass Index Since 1980: Systematic Analysis of Health Examination Surveys and Epidemiological Studies with 960 Country-Years and 9.1 Million Participants," *Lancet* 377, no. 9765 (February 12, 2011):557–67. Published electronically February 3, 2011.

8 R. Grucza et al., "The Emerging Link Between Alcoholism Link and Obesity in the US," *Archives of General Psychiatry* 67, no. 12 (2010):1301–8.

9 A. Gearhardt, "Food and Addiction: What It Is, How It Is Measured in Humans." http://www.youtube.com/watch?v=Y99bE-OG9r8.

10 American Heart Association's Nutrition, Physical Activity and Metabolism/Cardiovascular Disease Epidemiology and Prevention 2011 Scientific Sessions. http://www.medicalnewstoday.com/articles/220231.php.

11 N. Volkow and R. Wise, "How Can Drug Addiction Help Us Understand Obesity?" *Nature Neuroscience* 8, no. 5 (May 2005):555–60. Published electronically April 26, 2005. http://www.nature.com/neuro/journal/v8/n5/abs/nn1452.html.

12 http://www.hbo.com/addiction/thefilm/supplemental/624_nora_volkow.html.

13 J. A. Cummings et al., "Effects of a Selectively Bred Novelty-Seeking Phenotype on the Motivation to Take Cocaine in Male and Female Rats," *Biology of Sex Differences* 2, no. 1 (March 11, 2011):3. doi:10.1186/2042-6410-2-3.

14 http://newsfeed.time.com/2011/03/04/blair-river-heart-attack-grill-spokesman-dead-at-29-from-the-flu/.

15 http://www.hbo.com/addiction/thefilm/supplemental/624_nora_volkow.html.

16 Volkow and Wise, "How Can Drug Addiction Help Us Understand Obesity?"

17 F. H. Previc, "Dopamine and the Origins of Human Intelligence," *Brain and Cognition* 41, no. 3 (December 1999):299–350.

CHAPTER 2

1 N. Volkow and R. Wise, "How Can Drug Addiction Help Us Understand Obesity?" *Nature Neuroscience* 8, no. 5 (May 2005):555–60. Published electronically April 26, 2005. http://www.nature.com/neuro/journal/v8/n5/abs/nn1452.html.

2 J. A. Mennella, "Prenatal and Postnatal Flavor Learning by Human Infants," *Pediatrics* 107, no. 6 (June 2001):E88.

3 Z. Y. Ong and B. S. Muhlhausler, "Maternal 'Junk-Food' Feeding of Rat Dams Alters Food Choices and Development of the Mesolimbic Reward Pathway in the Offspring," *FASEB Journal* 25, no. 7 (July 2011):2167–79. doi:10.1096/fj.10-178392.

4 I. Sandovici et al., "Maternal Diet and Aging Alter the Epigenetic Control of a Promoter-Enhancer Interaction at the Hnf4a Gene in Rat Pancreatic Islets," *Proceedings of the National Academy of Sciences of the USA* 108, no. 13 (March 29, 2011):5449–54. Published electronically March 8, 2011.

5 J. A. Mennella, M. Y. Pepino, S. M. Lehmann-Castor, and L. M. Yourshaw, "Sweet Preferences and Analgesia during Childhood: Effects of Family History of Alcoholism and Depression," *Addiction* 105, no. 4 (April 2010):666–75. Published electronically February 9, 2010.

6 Ibid.

7 http://www.ewg.org/report/sugar_in_childrens_cereals/more_sugar.

8 K. Northstone et al., "Are Dietary Patterns in Childhood Associated with IQ at 8 Years of Age? A Population-Based Cohort Study," *Journal of Epidemiology and Community Health*. Published electronically February 7, 2011. http://jech.bmj.com/content/early/2011/01/21/jech.2010.111955.abstract.

9 L. Pryor, "Developmental Trajectories of Body Mass Index in Early Childhood and Their Risk Factors," *Archives of Pediatric and Adolescent Medicine* 165, no. 10 (2011):906–12.

10 J. M. Schwarz et al., "Early-Life Experience Decreases Drug-Induced Reinstatement of Morphine CPP in Adulthood via Microglial-Specific Epigenetic Programming of Anti-Inflammatory IL-10 Expression," *Journal of Neuroscience* 31, no. 49 (December 7, 2011):17835–47.

11 A. C. Grunseit et al., "Composite Measures Quantify Households' Obesogenic Potential and Adolescents' Risk Behaviors," *Pediatrics* 128, no. 2 (August 2011):e308–16.

12 S. S. Covington, "Women and Addiction: A Trauma-Informed Approach," *Journal of Psychoactive Drugs*, suppl. 5 (November 2008):377–85.

13 C. Liston et al., "Psychosocial Stress Reversibly Disrupts Prefrontal Processing and Attentional Control," *Proceedings of the National Academy of Sciences of the USA* 106, no. 3 (January 20, 2009):912–17. Published electronically January 12, 2009.

14 A. F. Arnsten, "Stress Signalling Pathways That Impair Prefrontal Cortex Structure and Function," *Nature Reviews Neuroscience* 10, no. 6 (June 2009):410–22.

15 K. Harmon, "Dopamine Determines Impulsive Behavior," *Scientific American*, July 29, 2010.

16 S. S. Lee et al., "Prospective Association of Childhood Attention-Deficit/Hyperactivity Disorder (ADHD) and Substance Use and Abuse/Dependence: A Meta-Analytic Review," *Clinical Psychology Review* 31, no. 3 (April 2011):328–41. Published electronically January 20, 2011.

17 C. Davis et al., "Evidence That 'Food Addiction' Is a Valid Phenotype of Obesity," *Appetite* 57, no. 3 (December 2011):711–17. Published electronically September 3, 2011.

18 http://whyquit.com/whyquit/LinksAAddiction.html.

19 R. A. Pretlow, "Addiction to Highly Pleasurable Food as a Cause of the Childhood Obesity Epidemic: A Qualitative Internet Study," *Eating Disorders* 19, no. 4 (July 2011):295–307. Published electronically June 21, 2011.

20 http://oyc.yale.edu/psychology/the-psychology-biology-and-politics-of-food/content/transcripts/transcript-6-culture-and-the-remarkable-plasticity.

21 D. V. Wang and J. Z. Tsien, "Convergent Processing of Both Positive and Negative Motivational Signals by the VTA Dopamine Neuronal Populations," *PLoS ONE* 6, no. 2 (February 15, 2011):e17047.

22 A. E. Kelley et al., "Restricted Daily Consumption of a Highly Palatable Food (Chocolate Ensure) Alters Striatal Enkephalin Gene Expression," *European Journal of Neuroscience* 18, no. 9 (November 2003):2592–98.

23 J. P. Thaler et al., "Obesity Is Associated with Hypothalamic Injury in Rodents and Humans," *Journal of Clinical Investigation* 122, no. 1 (January 3, 2012):153–62. Published electronically 2011 December 27, 2011. doi: 10.1172/JCI59660.

24 Volkow and Wise, "How Can Drug Addiction Help Us Understand Obesity?"

25 http://www.hbo.com/addiction/thefilm/supplemental/624_nora_volkow.html.

CHAPTER 3

1 http://publications.ki.se/jspui/bitstream/10616/37904/1/thesis.pdf.

2 M. Lenoir and F. Serre, "Intense Sweetness Surpasses Cocaine Reward," *PLoS ONE* 2, no. 8 (August 2007).

3 M. A. Parvaz et al., "Structural Integrity of the Prefrontal Cortex Modulates Electrocortical Sensitivity to Reward," *Journal of Cognitive Neuroscience*. Published electronically November 18, 2011.

4 P. M. Johnson and P. J. Kenny, "Dopamine D2 Receptors in Addiction-Like Reward Dysfunction and Compulsive Eating in Obese Rats," *Nature Neuroscience* 13, no. 5 (May 2010):635–41. Published electronically March 28, 2010. doi:10.1038/nn.2519.

5 K. Harmon, "Addicted to Fat: Overeating May Alter the Brain as Much as Hard Drugs," *Scientific American*, March 28, 2010. http://www.scientificamerican.com/article.cfm?id=addicted-to-fat-eating.

6 C. S. Soon et al., "Unconscious Determinants of Free Decisions in the Human Brain," *Nature Neuroscience* 11 (2008):543–45. Published electronically April 13, 2008. doi:10.1038/nn.2112.

32 C. M. Hansen, J. E. Leklem, and L. T. Miller, "Vitamin B-6 Status of Women with a Constant Intake of Vitamin B-6 Changes with Three Levels of Dietary Protein," *Journal of Nutrition* 126, no. 7 (1996):1891–901.

33 G. M. Timmerman, "Restaurant Eating in Nonpurge Binge-Eating Women," *Western Journal of Nursing Research* 28, no. 7 (November 2006):811–24; discussion 825–30.

34 A. Sánchez-Villegas et al., "Dietary Fat Intake and the Risk of Depression: The SUN Project," *PLoS ONE* 6, no. 1 (January 26, 2011):e16268.

35 J. Q. Purnell et al., "Brain Functional Magnetic Resonance Imaging Response to Glucose and Fructose Infusions in Humans," *Diabetes, Obesity, and Metabolism* 13, no. 3 (March 2011):229–34. doi: 10.1111/j.1463-1326.2010.01340.x.

36 http://www.nytimes.com/2011/02/20/health/20monkey.html.

37 P. G. MacRae et al., "Endurance Training Effects on Striatal D2 Dopamine Receptor Binding and Striatal Dopamine Metabolites in Presenescent Older Rats," *Psychopharmacology* 92, no. 2 (1987):236–40.

38 http://johnratey.typepad.com/blog/2008/04/third-age-healt.html.

39 M. S. Buchowski et al., "Aerobic Exercise Training Reduces Cannabis Craving and Use in Non-Treatment Seeking Cannabis-Dependent Adults," *PLoS ONE* 6, no. 3 (March 8, 2011):e17465.

40 L. A. Conlay, L. A. Sabounjian, and R. J. Wurtman, "Exercise and Neuromodulators: Choline and Acetylcholine in Marathon Runners," *International Journal of Sports Medicine* 13, suppl. 1 (October 1992):S141–42.

41 J. Crespo et al., "Nucleus Accumbens Core Acetylcholine Is Preferentially Activated During Acquisition of Drug- vs Food-Reinforced Behavior," *Neuropsychopharmacology* 42 (2008):3213–20. Published electronically April 16, 2008. doi:10.1038/npp.2008.48. http://www.nature.com/npp/journal/v33/n13/full/npp200848a.html.

42 K. Erickson et al., "Exercise Training Increases Size of Hippocampus and Improves Memory," *Proceedings of the National Academy of Sciences of the USA*. Published electronically January 31, 2011. doi: 10.1073/pnas.1015950108.

43 Smith et al., "Aerobic Exercise Decreases the Positive-Reinforcing Effects of Cocaine."

44 B. Leuner, E. R. Glasper, and E. Gould, "Sexual Experience Promotes Adult Neurogenesis in the Hippocampus Despite an Initial Elevation in Stress Hormones," *PLoS ONE* 5, no. 7 (July 14, 2010):e11597.

45 M. Chee, "Sleep Deprivation Alters Valuation Signals in the Ventromedial Prefrontal Cortex," *Frontiers in Behavioral Neuroscience* 5 (2011):70.

CHAPTER 6

1 T. W. Kjaer, et al., "Increased Dopamine Tone During Meditation-Induced Change of Consciousness," *Brain Research Cognitive Brain Research* 13, no. 2 (April 2002):255–59.

2 Ibid.

3 T. Durazzo, et al., "Cortical Thickness, Surface Area, and Volume of the Brain Reward System in Alcohol Dependence: Relationships to Relapse and Extended Abstinence," *Alcoholism: Clinical and Experimental Research* (2011). doi: 10.1111/j.1530-0277.2011.01452.x.

4 J. Hooper, "Meditation Nation," Details, September 2011. http://www.details.com/culture-trends/critical-eye/201109/transcendental-meditation-pure-consciousness.

5 http://www.nytimes.com/2011/03/20/fashion/20TM.html?pagewanted=2.

6 B. K. Hölzel et al., "Mindfulness Practice Leads to Increases in Regional Brain Gray Matter Density," *Psychiatry Research* 191, no. 1 (January 30, 2011):36–43. Published electronically November 10, 2010.

7 M. A. Noonan et al., "Reduction of Adult Hippocampal Neurogenesis Confers Vulnerability in an Animal Model of Cocaine Addiction," *Journal of Neuroscience* 30, no. 1 (January 6, 2010):304–15.

8 G. Riva et al., "Is Severe Obesity a Form of Addiction? Rationale, Clinical Approach, and Controlled Clinical Trial," *Cyberpsychology and Behavior* 9, no. 4 (August 2006):457–79.

9 B. Knauper et al., "Fruitful Plans: Adding Targeted Mental Imagery to Implementation Intentions Increases Fruit Consumption," *Psychology and Health* 26, no. 5 (May 2011):601–17. Published electronically February 18, 2011.

10 D. V. Wang and J. Z. Tsien, "Convergent Processing of Both Positive and Negative Motivational Signals by the VTA Dopamine Neuronal Populations," *PLoS ONE* 6, no. 2 (February 15, 2011):e17047.

11 T. Hare, "Focusing Attention on the Health Aspects of Foods Changes Value Signals in vmPFC and Improves Dietary Choice," *Journal of Neuroscience* 31, no. 30 (July 27, 2011):11077–87.

12 W. Bickel, "Remember the Future: Working Memory Training Decreases Delay Discounting Among Stimulant Addicts," *Biological Psychiatry* 69 (2011):260–65.

13 M. Yogo and S. Fujihara, "Working Memory Capacity Can Be Improved by Expressive Writing: A Randomized Experiment in a Japanese Sample," *British Journal of Health Psychology* 13, no. 1 (February 2008):77–80.

14 F. Zeidan et al., "Mindfulness Meditation Improves Cognitions: Evidence of Brief Mental Training," *Consciousness and Cognition* 19, no. 2 (June 2010):597–605.

15 E. Stice et al., "Weight Gain Is Associated with Reduced Striatal Response to Palatable Food," *Journal of Neuroscience* 30, no. 39 (September 29, 2010):13105–9.

16 E. Stice et al., "Relation of Obesity to Consummatory and Anticipatory Food Reward," *Physiology and Behavior* 97, no. 5 (July 14, 2009):551–60. Published electronically March 27, 2009.

17 B. Knauper et al., "Fruitful Plans."

18 S. Wang, "Improvement in Chewing Activity Reduces Energy Intake in One Meal and Modulates Plasma Gut Hormone Concentrations in Obese and Lean Young Chinese Men," *American Journal of Clinical Nutrition* 94 (2011):709–16.

19 http://nutritiondata.self.com/foods-000087000000000000000.html.

20 B. Hoebel, N. Avena, and P. Rada, "Accumbens Dopamine-Acetylcholine Balance in Approach and Avoidance," *Current Opinion in Pharmacology* 7, no. 6 (December 2007):617–27. doi:10.1016/j.coph.2007.10.014.

21 N. Sandstrom, "Prenatal Choline Supplementation Increases NGF Levels in the Hippocampus and Frontal Cortex of Young and Adult Rats," *Brain Research* 947 (2002):9–16.

22 R. Tees, "The Influences of Rearing Environment and Neonatal Choline Dietary Supplementation on Spatial Learning and Memory in Adult Rats," *Behavioural Brain Research* 105, no. 2 (1999):173–88.

23 https://www.uleth.ca/dspace/bitstream/handle/10133/222/MR03034.pdf?sequence=3.

24 D. D. Rasmusson, "The Role of Acetylcholine in Cortical Synaptic Plasticity," *Behavioural Brain Research* 115, no. 2 (November 2000):205–18.

25 R. K. McNamara, "Docosahexaenoic Acid Supplementation Increases Prefrontal Cortex Activation During Sustained Attention in Healthy Boys: A Placebo-Controlled, Dose-Ranging, Functional Magnetic Resonance Imaging Study," *American Journal of Clinical Nutrition* 91, no. 4 (April 2010):1060–67.

26 R. A. Johnson et al., "Hippocampal Brain-Derived Neurotrophic Factor but Not Neurotrophin-3 Increases More in Mice Selected for Increased Voluntary Wheel Running," *Neuroscience* 121, no. 1 (2003):1–7.

27 http://www.ergotron.com/portals/0/literature/other/english/ACSM_SittingTime.pdf.

28 M. A. Smith et al., "Aerobic Exercise Decreases the Positive-Reinforcing Effects of Cocaine," *Drug and Alcohol Dependence* 98, no. (1–2 (November 1, 2008):129–35. Published electronically June 27, 2008.

29 M. J. Berry et al., "A Comparison between Two Forms of Aerobic Dance and Treadmill Running," *Medicine and Science in Sports and Exercise* 24, no. 8 (August 1992):946–51.

30 J. P. Little et al., "Low-Volume High-Intensity Interval Training Reduces Hyperglycemia and Increases Muscle Mitochondrial Capacity in Patients with Type 2 Diabetes," *Journal of Applied Physiology* 111, no. 6 (December 2011):1554–60.

31 T. Liu-Ambrose et al., "Resistance Training and Executive Functions: A 12-Month Randomized Controlled Trial," *Archives of Internal Medicine* 170, no. 2 (January 25, 2010):170–78.

32 J. T. Ciccolo, "Resistance Training as an Aid to Standard Smoking Cessation Treatment: A Pilot Study," *Nicotine and Tobacco Research* 13, no. 8 (August 2011):756–60. Published electronically April 18, 2011.

33 P. Srikanthan and A. S. Karlamangla, "Relative Muscle Mass Is Inversely Associated with Insulin Resistance and Prediabetes. Findings from the Third National Health and Nutrition Examination Survey," *Journal of Clinical Endocrinology and Metabolism* 96, no. 9 (September 2011):2898–903. Published electronically July 21, 2011.

34 R. D. Badgaiyan, "Dopamine Is Released in the Striatum during Human Emotional Processing," *Neuroreport* 21, no 18 (December 29, 2010):1172–76.

35 B. J. Park, "The Physiological Effects of Shinrin-yoku (Taking in the Forest Atmosphere or Forest Bathing): Evidence from Field Experiments in 24 Forests across Japan," *Environmental Health and Preventive Medicine* 15, no. 1 (January 2010):18–26.

36 R. Kanter, "Trees, Green Space, and Human Well-Being," *Environmental Almanac* radio show, Thursday, July 7, 2005. http://lhhl.illinois.edu/media/2005.07_kanter.htm.

37 S. N. Young, "How to Increase Serotonin in the Human Brain Without Drugs," *Journal of Psychiatry and Neuroscience* 32, no. 6 (November 2007):394–99. http://www.ncbi.nlm.nih.gov/pmc/articles/PMC2077351.

38 http://www.cet.org/eng/DayLightSimulator_ENG.html.

39 M. J. Koepp et al., "Evidence for Striatal Dopamine Release During a Video Game," *Nature* 393, no. 6682 (May 21, 1998):266–68.

40 M. Miyachi et al., "METs in Adults While Playing Active Video Games: A Metabolic Chamber Study," *Medicine and Science in Sports and Exercise* 42, no. 6 (June 2010):1149–53.

41 J. R. Worley, S. N. Rogers, and R. R. Kraemer. "Metabolic Responses to Wii Fit Video Games at Different Game Levels," *Journal of Strength and Conditioning Research* 25, no. 3 (March 2011):689–93.

42 D. Bavelier, C. S. Green, and M. W. Dye, "Children, Wired: for Better and for Worse," *Neuron* 67, no. 5 (September 9, 2010):692–701.

43 E. Nofzinger, "Frontal Cerebral Thermal Transfer as a Treatment for Insomnia: A Dose-Ranging Study." *Journal of Sleep and Sleep Disorders Research*, abstract 0534, Volume 34, 2011, Abstract Supplement.

CHAPTER 7

1 G. Leonard, *Mastery: The Keys to Success and Long-Term Fulfillment* (New York: Dutton, 1991).

2 http://www.fi.edu/learn/brain/proteins.html; L. Bäckman et al., "Age-Related Cognitive Deficits Mediated by Changes in the Striatal Dopamine System," *American Journal of Psychiatry* 157, no. 4 (April 2000):635–37.

3 J. Proietto, "Long-Term Persistence of Hormonal Adaptations to Weight Loss," *New England Journal of Medicine* 365, no. 17 (October 27, 2011):1586–96.

4 R. L. Batterham, "Pancreatic Polypeptide Reduces Appetite and Food Intake in Humans," *Journal of Clinical Endocrinology and Metabolism* 88, no. 8 (August 2003):3989–92.

5 R. J. Joseph et al., "The Neurocognitive Connection Between Physical Activity and Eating Behaviour," *Obesity Reviews* 12, no. 10 (October 2011):800–12. Published electronically June 16, 2011. doi: 10.1111/j.1467-789X.2011.00893.x.

6 D. V. Wang and J. Z. Tsien, "Convergent Processing of Both Positive and Negative Motivational Signals by the VTA Dopamine Neuronal Populations," *PLoS ONE* 6, no. 2 (February 15, 2011):e17047.

7 http://www.thenakedscientists.com/HTML/articles/article/dalyacolumn6.htm.

8 http://www.thenakedscientists.com/HTML/articles/article/dalyacolumn6.htm.

9 http://www.psychologytoday.com/blog/the-playing-field/200803/the-addictive-nature-adrenaline-sport.

10 F. G. Ashby FG, A. M. Isen AM, and A. U. Turken, "A Neuropsychological Theory of Positive Affect and Its Influence on Cognition," *Psychological Review* 106, no. 3 (July 1999):529–50.

11 M. Pagano et al., "Alcoholics Anonymous-Related Helping and the Helper Therapy Principle," *Alcoholism Treatment Quarterly* 29, no. 1 (January 2011):23–24.

12 http://greatergood.berkeley.edu/article/item/the_helpers_high.

13 T. Eagle et al., "Health Status and Behavior Among Middle-School Children in a Midwest Community: What Are the Underpinnings of Childhood Obesity?" *American Heart Journal* 160, no. 6 (December 2010):1185–89.

14 http://jhfowler.ucsd.edu/friends_drd4_and_political_ideology.pdf.

15 S. Carson, "The Unleashed Mind: Why Creative People Are Eccentric," *Scientific American Mind*, April 14, 2011.

16 I. Fried et al., "Increased Dopamine Release in the Human Amygdala During Performance of Cognitive Tasks," *Nature Neuroscience* 4, no. 2 (February 2001):201–6.

17 F. McNab et al., "Changes in Cortical Dopamine D1 Receptor Binding Associated with Cognitive Training," *Science* 323, no. 5915 (February 6, 2009):800–802.

18 H. R. Brattbakk et al., "Balanced Caloric Macronutrient Composition Downregulates Immunological Gene Expression in Human Blood Cells-Adipose Tissue Diverges," *OMICS*. Published electronically June 16. 2011.

19 INTERHEART investigative team, "The Effect of Chromosome 9p21 Variants on Cardiovascular Disease May Be Modified by Dietary Intake: Evidence from a Case/Control and a Prospective Study," *PLoS Medicine* 8, no. 10 (October 2011):e1001106. Published electronically October 11, 2011.

20 http://learn.genetics.utah.edu/content/epigenetics/nutrition.

21 http://dashinghealth.com/tag/methyl-donor.

22 http://www.umm.edu/altmed/articles/s-adenosylmethionine-000324.htm.

23 http://www.nal.usda.gov/fnic/foodcomp/Data/Other/IFT2004_Betaine.pdf.

24 J. K. Blusztajn and T. J. Mellott, "Choline Nutrition Programs Brain Development via DNA and Histone Methylation," *Central Nervous System Agents in Medicinal Chemistry*. Published electronically April 2, 2012.

25 http://lpi.oregonstate.edu/infocenter/othernuts/choline.

26 http://www.academicjournals.org/ajmr/PDF/Pdf2009/Nov/Rattanachaikunsopon%20and%20Phumkhachorn.pdf.

27 http://lpi.oregonstate.edu/infocenter/phytochemicals/resveratrol.

28 http://ods.od.nih.gov/factsheets/vitaminb6/#h3.

29 S. Witherly, *Why Humans Like Junk Food: The Inside Story on Why You Like Your Favorite Foods, the Cuisine Secrets of Top Chefs, and How to Improve Your Own Cooking Without a Recipe!* (Lincoln, NE: iUniverse, 2007).

30 A. Goel, "Novel Evidence for Curcumin-Induced DNA Methylation Changes in Colon Cancer Cells," *Gastroenterology* 138, no. 5, Suppl. 1 (May 2010):S–349. http://download.journals.elsevierhealth.com/pdfs/journals/0016-5085/PIIS0016508510616083.pdf.

31 J. U. Adams, "Obesity, Epigenetics, and Gene Regulation," *Nature Education* 1, no. 1 (2008).

32 http://blog.case.edu/think/2011/02/17/apes_shed_pounds_while_doubling_calories_cwru_researcher_finds.

33 http://www.eurekalert.org/pub_releases/2011-02/cwru-asp021611.php.

34 J. Barton and J. Pretty, "What Is the Best Dose of Nature and Green Exercise for Improving Mental Health? A Multi-Study Analysis," *Environmental Science and Technology* 44, no. 10 (May 15, 2010):3947–55.

35 K. N. Boutelle et al., "Two Novel Treatments to Reduce Overeating in Overweight Children: A Randomized Controlled Trial," *Journal of Consulting and Clinical Psychology* 79, no. 6 (December 2011):759–71.

36 L. Cao et al., "White to Brown Fat Phenotypic Switch Induced by Genetic and Environmental Activation of a Hypothalamic-Adipocyte Axis," *Cell Metabolism* 14, no. 3 (September 7, 2011):324–38.

37 P. Boström et al., "A PGC1–Dependent Myokine That Drives Brown-Fat-Like Development of White Fat and Thermogenesis," *Nature* 481, no. 7382 (January 12, 2012):463–68. doi: 10.1038/nature10777

38 C. L. Davis et al., "Exercise Improves Executive Function and Achievement and Alters Brain Activation in Overweight Children: A Randomized, Controlled Trial," *Health Psychology* 30(1 (January 2011):91–98.

39 N. D. Volkow et al., "Sleep Deprivation Decreases Binding of [11C]Raclopride to Dopamine D2/D3 Receptors in the Human Brain," *Journal of Neuroscience* 28, no. 34 (August 20, 2008):8454–61.

40 H. Myrseth et al., "A Comparison of Impulsivity and Sensation Seeking in Pathological Gamblers and Skydivers," *Scandinavian Journal of Psychology.* Published electronically September 19, 2011. doi: 10.1111/j.1467-9450.2011.00917.x.

CHAPTER 8

1 M. M. Karnani et al., "Activation of Central Orexin/Hypocretin Neurons by Dietary Amino Acids," *Neuron* 72, no. 4 (November 17, 2011):616–29.

2 http://www.menshealth.com/mhlists/simple_steps_to_live_longer/index.php.

3 NYC Department of Health and Mental Hygiene, *Eat Street Smart.* http://www.nyc.gov/html/doh/downloads/pdf/cdp/greencarts-brochure-online.pdf. Accessed January 31, 2011.

4 http://www.diabetesselfmanagement.com/pdfs/DSM0309_036.pdf.

APPENDIX A

1 A. N. Gearhardt, W. R. Corbin, and K. D. Brownell, "Preliminary Validation of the Yale Food Addiction Scale," *Appetite* 52, no. 2 (April 2009):430–36. Published electronically December 11, 2008.

APPENDIX F

1 http://sghealthyapps.challenge.gov/updates/178.

Acknowledgments

Over the course of a decade, I waited impatiently for the critical mass of neuroscience to pave the way for the writing of this book. When at last that day arrived, I called upon my intrepid team to get the ball rolling. Fascinated with the new science, my agent Andrea Barzvi was my ever-present guide from proposal to finished manuscript. Her passion and belief in the importance of the book never wavered and for that I'm deeply grateful to her and to ICM.

Writing this book was quite a journey and one that could never have happened without Mariska van Aalst by my side. Smart and savvy, she set about the task of wading through reams of research, organizing data, and finally wordsmithing it into powerful prose. I will never be able to thank her enough for her encouragement, expertise, and most of all, the endless supply of smiles, laughs, and friendship. Mariska is a diamond in my life's tiara.

My Rodale team was stellar. Sincere thanks go out to David Zinczenko and Steve Perrine for their energetic support. My editor, Ursula Cary, ever the calm in any deadline storm, was the queen of the gentle reminder. I will always cherish the memory of the infamous cupcake photo shoot she gladly finessed (along with the talented Amy King) for the cover. I'd also like to thank Nancy Bailey, Faith Hague, and Susan Hindman for their efforts to perfect every page.

Writing a book with so much groundbreaking science provided the opportunity to meet extraordinary scientists like Dr. Nora Volkow, director of the National Institute of Drug Abuse. During our interview, I realized I was in the presence of a brilliant revolutionary in neuroscience. I'm deeply grateful to Drs. Mike Pazin and Vivien Bonazzi from the NIH's National Human Genome Research Institute, who helped tutor me in the emerging field of epigenetics, another science revolution in the making. I also owe a debt of gratitude to Duke University's Dr. Randy Jirtle for providing me with his history-making Agouti mice research and pictures.

A special word of deep gratitude goes out to the amazing SPE (Sanitas Per Escam, or Health Through Nutrition) culinary nutritionists who created the food plans and recipes that, with every bite, guarantee you'll reclaim your brain's reward system. Natalia Hancock and Andrea Canada spent hours tirelessly crafting the Healthy Fix cuisine, with the support of SPE founders Manu Verstaeten and Nil Sonmez. I cannot wait for the world to have a taste and truly savor health!

This book was an opportunity to collaborate with many friends and colleagues: Biggest Loser celebrity Tara Costa; Dr. Jim Hill of the National Weight Control Registry; Dr. Norman Rosenthal, *New York Times* bestselling author of *Transcendence;* Dr. David Kessler, former FDA commissioner and author of *The End of Overeating,* Dr. Kelly Brownell, senior editor of the first textbook on food and addiction; Yale University food addiction researcher Dr. Ashley Gearhardt; the professionals I interviewed at the American Society of Addiction Medicine; Nancy Clark, sports nutritionist extraordinaire; US Surgeon General Dr. Regina Benjamin; Zumba CEO Alberto Perlman; Dr. Michael Smith and the WebMD team; Bob Roth, executive director of the David Lynch Foundation; Curves cofounders Diane and Gary Heavin; Anytime Fitness cofounders Chuck Runyon and Dave Mortensen; Jim Whitehead and the ACSM gang; Dr. Paul Terpeluk, Cleveland Clinic addiction expert; Deborah Szekely, founder of the Golden Door; and Miraval CEO Michael Tompkins. Writing a book is one goal, but getting the word out is the challenge that Sandi Mendelson and her amazing PR professionals are more than up to.

I'm blessed with an embarrassment of riches in my friends and kindred spirits, my Team Peeke: Naomi Henderson, Judy Fitzpatrick, Kay Kirkpatrick, Linda and John Solheim, Rebecca Krisman, Mary Lou and Chuck Gervie, Bob Madigan, Jane Pemberton, Augie Nieto, Karen Strong, Jason Mintz, Tim Friel, Brian Averi, Richel D'Ambra, Frances Kuffel, John Lydon, Father Jeremy Harrington. Under the guidance of TM teachers Mario Orsatti and Linda Mainquist, I regularly medicated with meditation to stay focused and centered in the eye of the publishing storm. To maintain my sanity, I had to have a nonwriting goal—running the Boston marathon! Olympic marathoner Jeff Galloway patiently guided my ever-interrupted training, his calming words resonating in my head as I sprinted to the finish line. Danny Dreyer helped me find the "chi" in my running as well as my writing.

Eternal thanks to my family for putting up with my endless days and nights sequestered in the writing cave. Mark, Art, and Sheila were ever present to offer me love and support through computer mishaps, power outages, and a fractured foot. I shared the highs and the lows with Desiree, my soul mate sis and a lifesaver. Bros Ray and Ted hung in there with me. I turned to four-legged companionship with 5-0, my black-as-night Serbian German Shepherd who never left my side as I hit the pavement every day, running and walking off daily stresses.

For all of these remarkable folks in my life, I am deeply grateful and forever blessed.

Index

Boldface page references indicate photos or illustrations. Underscored references indicate tables or boxed text.